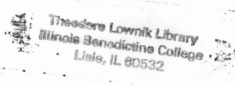

DOCTORS
ARE
GODS

DOCTORS
ARE
GODS

~

CORRUPTION
AND UNETHICAL PRACTICES
IN THE
MEDICAL PROFESSION

David Jacobsen
AND
Eric D. Jacobsen

THUNDER'S MOUTH PRESS
NEW YORK

174.2
J17d

First edition
First printing, 1994

Published by
Thunder's Mouth Press
632 Broadway, 7th Floor
New York, NY 10012

Library of Congress Cataloging-in-Publication Data

Jacobsen, David.
    Doctors are Gods : corruption and unethical practices in the
  medical profession / David Jacobsen and Eric D. Jacobsen.—1st ed.
      p.   cm.
    ISBN 1-56025-070-4 : $22.95
    1. Medical ethics.   2. Medical personnel—Malpractice.
  I. Jacobsen, Eric.   II. Title.
  R724.J32   1994
  174'.2—dc20   93-46716
                                                        CIP

Printed in the United States of America

Distributed by
Publishers Group West
4065 Hollis Street
Emeryville, CA 94608
(800) 788-3123

To our Mother and Grandmother, Anna Madsenbeck Jacobsen, who blessed us with her wisdom, courage, love and discipline. She also blessed thousands through a lifetime of being a nurse.

Acknowledgments

During our many years in hospital management, many people have passed through our lives. Some negatively affected us by their private agendas for greed and ego glorification. It would have been easy, and at times tempting, to just walk away from health care. But we were fortunate men to have friends of quality whose values sustained us through the dark times.

Manzoor Massey, PhD, MPH, must be thanked for providing material on the evolution of patient-physician relationships and how to select a good physician. An expert in medical sociology, he provided the academic balance to the story of a health care system in need of healing.

Dean of Medicine, Dr. Raja Khuri; Director of Nursing Gladys Mouro; and Controller, Joe Cicippio are saints who managed to keep the American University of Beirut Medical Center together when society crossed that narrow line between civilization and barbarism. Dr. John Mohler and his wife, Mary Ellen, have been a constant source of inspiration and emulation. David's first boss in health care, Alfred Thomas, was a model of personal honesty who never surrendered to the political system. Dr. Paul Hoagland, an internist from Pasadena, California, was the professional and ethical standard to measure all physicians. To paraphrase President Kennedy's comments about Thomas Jefferson, the only time that the collective wisdom of all hospital executives gathered together in one room could be exceeded would be when Samuel "Sollie" Sedell dines alone. Sollie has been a leader, mentor and true friend to so many of us in health care. These role models provided the spirit to make this book possible.

Eric would like to thank his four-year-old daughter, Erika Ann, who patiently sacrificed our regular bedtime stories to allow Daddy the necessary time to transcribe and compile the manuscript. And to his wife, Cathy, who was the best benefit of his years of working in the medical field.

Our agent Frank Weimann served us well. We are also grateful to Joan Fucillo, our editor, for her encouragement and wise counsel, and the commitment of publisher Neil Ortenberg, who enabled us to make this story public.

Contents

Introduction

"The competent physician, before he attempts to give medicine to his patient, makes himself acquainted not only with the disease which he wishes to cure, but also with the habits and constitution of the sick man."

Cicero: *De oratore, II,* c 80 BC

Until recently, these words have been the backbone of the healing arts. From prehistoric witch doctors to ancient Greek physicians to medieval priest-doctors to the physicians of the twentieth century, the personal relationship between the practitioner and the patient has been the foundation for the practice of medicine. And when all the technology and financial considerations are put aside, the successful practice of medicine is still the healing of one person by another.

A social animal, man seems to have a genetic need for personal relationships, and other things being equal, a friend makes a better physician than a stranger. But now it does seem that where health-care providers were once our friends, they are now strangers. In the 1930s and 40s, the doctor who delivered us was our family's physician—our obstetrician, pediatrician, internist, surgeon, family counselor. He lived and practiced from his home in our neighborhood, and he belonged to our social and economic community. He had a stake in our lives; he spent time with us. Likewise, if you were hospitalized, the nurse spent more time with you than with paperwork or machines. She held your hand. She had time for conversation. The local pharmacist was your friend. His store's soda fountain was the social center of Main Street. Not only did he mix your medicine, he made your tuna sandwich and chocolate malt.

Now six-lane highways speed nurses and technicians to work at hospitals outside of their own communities. Physicians seem to pass through the examination room so quickly that patients may think they're suffering from blurred vision. Health care has become mobile and impersonal and the neighborhood medical facility is disappearing. The personal relationships of yesterday have been replaced by the technology, indifference and the bottom line of big business. Government bureaucracy and corporate monsters spread their control and influence into every sector of health care. And now it seems that competition will be destroyed and there will be even fewer health-care providers. We find ourselves longing for what has been. We look once again to assimilate into the health-care "community."

With the 1990 national elections, the weaknesses of our health-care system were brought to the forefront of public awareness. Those of us who have practical experience working in the health-care industry were generally pleased to see the attention. However, we also noticed that it was the press and the politicians who were defining the issues, not health-care professionals, as these well-intentioned and well-motivated social scientists began making their elaborate and complicated suggestions for reforming the system. While they've raised many valid points, we are worried about the direction of the debate. Too often, our conceptions of health care are based on dramatized television shows or public opinion polls, none of which are appropriate means for comprehending complex problems. We cannot allow decisions that will affect us and future generations to be based on twenty seconds of sound bite, reactionary public opinion polls, political rhetoric or PAC money.

What has caused us the greatest concern in the year-long health care debate has been the issues that *aren't* being discussed. The current proposals cover a wide range of health-care options, but they all fail to address the most basic problem in the system— its inability to uncover, police and correct the unethical, fraudulent and immoral practices of a small percentage of health-care providers.

We've all heard of or experienced doctor and hospital horror stories. These range from the mundane (bad coffee and slow service) to the frightening: switched patients and wrongful deaths. That's what the public knows. But what the public doesn't see, what the industry has kept hidden, what nobody really seems to want to talk about, is the daily fraudulent and unscrupulous actions that go unchecked and unpoliced. While the percentage of physicians and health-care providers involved in fraud is quite small, the huge amounts of money flowing through the system, coupled with the health-care recipient's inherent dependency and vulnerability, has made this the single greatest issue affecting sky-rocketing costs—to the tune of tens of billions of dollars annually. If we want to pinpoint the source of our health-care crisis, that's the place to begin. Yet, if this is true, why hasn't the issue been addressed? The answer is simple: the general public and its political leadership do not understand the actual organization of and daily practice of medicine.

This book grew out of a kind of town hall meeting for health-care insiders. In over a hundred interviews conducted over a period of a year, we elicited comments and insights from doctors, nurses, administrators, technologists, pharmacists, nurse practitioners, hospital support staff, trustees, medical equipment and supplies sales representatives, legal investigators, health-care attorneys, social workers, health-care educators, insurance providers, and executives of hospital and medical professional organizations. These are the people of health care, the hardworking daily providers, who have not had an outlet to express their opinions. We purposely did not interview those people quoted daily in the news media—lobbyists, leaders in national organizations, politicians or CEOs (with the exception of hospital administrators), because we wanted to provide a forum for health-care workers, the majority of whom silently and efficiently extend their healing touch with compassion and care. To our knowledge, none of those we spoke with had talked with anyone from President Clinton's task force on health care.

The impetus for this project was our concern about the future of health care in this country, which was grounded in our personal experience in the industry. David Jacobsen is a seasoned CEO/Administrator with thirty years' of hospital management experience. David has served in hospitals ranging in size from one hundred to six hundred beds in both urban and rural communities, including religious, not-for-profit, investor-owned, government and university. Over the years David has participated in thousands of medical committee meetings and has dealt with thousands of physicians and other health-care professionals in every aspect of medicine. Eric Jacobsen has seen the industry from a different perspective, having six years' experience in ancillary services and four more with an independent medical equipment service and sales company. Eric left the industry six years ago but has maintained an insider's attention to the workings of and the problems of health-care delivery. Together, we have nearly half a century of expertise in health care and a vast array of contacts in all aspects of health care. As we began the process of searching out contributors, we called upon many of those contacts, but at the conclusion of our interviews we were somewhat surprised but gratified to discover that the majority of those we spoke with had been previously unknown to us on either a personal or professional basis.

The interviewing process was simple. When we first made contact, we explained our purpose as threefold: to educate the general public as to how the health-care industry really works; to give each participant the opportunity to identify what they thought were the biggest problem areas in health care, especially those which they thought were being ignored in the current debate; and finally, to offer their solutions. We didn't show up for these interviews with a list of questions. Instead, we attempted to say as little as possible and give the interviewees control over the course of the conversation. We acknowledged immediately to them that we were not trained journalists and never attempted to pass ourselves off as such.

Since participation in our town hall was presented as a chance to discuss the failings of our health-care system freely, directly, and honestly, those who spoke with us were extended anonymity to allow them the freedom to share their insights and opinions without fear of retaliation or recrimination. Perhaps because of this freedom, a darker side of medicine did emerge. Indeed, some comments may strike the reader as strong or vindictive. However, this seemed to us to indicate the real frustration many of these people had with the misconceptions and false expectations of the public; the system's failure to police abuses, which only an insider would be aware of; their own inability to prevent or rectify these abuses; and their sense of bitterness at a system that they saw as preventing them from doing their jobs—providing health care.

As editors of these conversations, it has been our task to identify the dominant themes cited by those who spoke with us and to group their comments into a readable text. While there was a wide variety of opinions, one theme was apparent from the outset: health care reform is inevitable. Along with this acknowledgment came an almost universally expressed hope that reform does not destroy the greatest health-care system in the world by sacrificing its greatest asset—the people who work in it. And we agree. We were constantly impressed by those we met, particularly by the altruistic spirit motivating each one. One of our hopes is that this book will serve as a defense of the good people in medicine.

While many of the comments focus on the problems in health care, we believe that seventy percent of health-care providers give far more than they receive in return—these are your friends and neighbors. Twenty-five percent are sheep who will follow any leader who happens to be present, good or evil. Five percent are incompetent, negligent, drug impaired, unscrupulous, immoral or unethical, and when that five percent is in charge of the sheep, that is when fraud and abuse abound. That small number, when allowed to control the sheep, is responsible for much of the financial trouble in health care.

What has allowed these breaches in health care ethics to occur? When asked, most spoke of the rift that has grown between provider and patient. It's as if there has been a slow, strong current of change that has worn away the landscape of health care, leading us downstream against our will. In the last fifty years, technical and therapeutic medical advances have exceeded all those of previously recorded history but something has gone terribly wrong—the system has lost the personal relationship that mankind expects and needs from its medical providers.

In the course of preparing this book, we found that some of our preconceptions were affirmed and others modified. While we don't agree with everything that's contained in these pages, we do hope it will serve as a catalyst for serious thought by the reader, who will then formulate his own opinions. We began from a desire to make a contribution to the debate currently before Congress and the nation, and it is our hope that the words of the health-care professionals we spoke with will help spark effective reform. Not reform based solely on financial considerations, but one grounded on a foundation of human trust and care. We hope that in the course of reading these personal comments, the humanness of our health-care system does not discourage the reader. Rather, we hope that the reader is encouraged by that notion, because humanness is the very thing that comforts and heals the sick. Medicine is not a divine art. Doctors are not gods. Technology is not the ultimate answer to every disease, ailment and condition. If reform is inevitable, then let's address the issues head-on. Otherwise, reform will be ineffective and may only exacerbate the problems that are behind the increasing costs and decreasing quality of our health care.

1

THE EVOLUTION OF
THE GODS OF MEDICINE

*Until recent generations, medicine has been perceived as a voca-
tion possessing a direct connection to the Divine and this attitude
persists today. Whereas in the past the link has been seen as spiritual, now the doctor gains access to the Divine through the mys-
teries of science and technology. It is an awesome responsibility
that generates many unrealistic expectations, but for better or
worse, the medical practitioner still remains the blessed go-between, the arbiter between sickness and mortality and the supernatural powers of healing.*

*We spoke at length with an expert in medical sociology about
the evolution of this concept, and how it affects current doctor-
patient relations.*

It might be of value for me to give you some background on
doctor-patient relationships. I think to understand current physician-patient relationships, it's important to look back through
history, especially the early Greek era and during the Middle
Ages in Europe. With that knowledge, one can understand the
age-old involvement of the State in the art of healing, and its
influence on the doctor-patient relationship.

All of the evidence indicates that the doctor in these early cultures, while treating the patient, was mindful of his client's background. The doctor rarely offended the patient, and consequently, the patient was more cooperative and they enjoyed a very strong and favorable relationship.

In the Greek world, as today, a sick person sought medical help because of his desire to be healed. That hasn't changed. A physician, on the other hand, was motivated solely by his spirit of *philia*, love or friendship, to help the invalid, rather than by his economic interests.

According to Plato, where there is *philanthropia*, the love of man, there is *philotechnica*, the love of art. Included in that was the love of the medical art of healing. Thus, for the Greeks, the relationship between the doctor and patient based on *philia* provided the basis for the practice of medicine.

The Greeks believed in the supernatural origin of disease; however, they saw in their doctor a person in the place of a god, a supreme and powerful being with enormous magic powers to bring health and healing. The Greek patient's confidence in the art of healing was ultimately based on the religious and sacred prestige surrounding the various arts. The ancient Greeks believed in the origin of the arts as a theft from the gods and for some, the doctor became a real god figure. Thus centuries ago, doctors became gods in the minds of a few patients and their families.

And in fact, the payment that most ancient Greeks gave the physician was not strictly pecuniary. Financial compensation was secondary to an even more priceless possession—not worship, but honor. They saw the physician as an honorable man. Respect implies confidence, and the Greek doctor enjoyed his patient's confidence.

While a Greek patient's confidence in medicine inspired confidence in his doctor, the Greek belief that some diseases were mortal or incurable by necessity, kept the patient's expectations of his doctor's skills on a more realistic level. The physician had no power to heal every disease at all times. The Greek physician did not pretend to restore all dangerously altered sick bodies to perfect beauty, health and harmony.

The basis of the Hippocratic advice, drawn up in 400 BC, instructed doctors to gain and retain the patient's confidence and there was detailed advice concerning the physician's behavior toward patients. On entering a patient's room, the doctor was to bear in mind his manner of sitting, emotional makeup, arrangement of dress, decisive utterance, brevity of speech, composure, concentration, readiness to do what had to be done. The doctor was cautioned that in the performance of his duty he should not thwart the bond of friendship which exists between him and his patient.

Plato further instructed the Greek physician to employ verbal persuasion in order to individualize the treatment and gain the patient's confidence. Plato put forth his most fundamental principle that the doctor was to explain to the patient the nature of his illness, the course of treatment, and possible outcome. This would afford the patient the opportunity to have all of his questions answered. The doctor was not to prescribe for his patient until he first convinced the patient of the possible effectiveness of that course of action.

Plato pointed out to the doctor that the most effective way to persuade the patient in favor of the treatment was to acquire an adequate case history . . . in other words, listen to the patient, an art that has been lost through the centuries. Both Plato and Aristotle emphasized the necessity of adjusting medical treatment to the patient's history. The doctor needed to know as much about his patient as possible, because knowledge to the doctor was a major source of building a wholesome relationship with the patient.

Reputation was of great importance to the Greek physician. Medicine was an art—educated people engaged in medical studies without ever intending to practice medicine. There were no medical institutions as such. No license to practice medicine granted by the State or any organization was given to the physician until the Middle Ages. There was no guarantee that the individual who treated patients for a fee had any medical knowledge except his reputation.

A person who wanted to study medicine became the apprentice of a physician. He paid his fee and worked with the doctor for years. The apprentice carried the doctor's medical bag and observed and took notes while his master treated his patients. The more famous the master, the more favorable the reputation of the apprentice after he became a physician.

The Hippocratic doctor was advised not to be greedy and to take the economic status of his patient into consideration, even to the point of giving free services occasionally. Larger communities in need of medical services usually invited a doctor and appointed him as the municipal physician and paid him an annual salary, which was raised through a special tax.

The doctor-patient relationship was the central issue in the practice of medicine in the early Greek era, and the doctor and patient did enjoy a very strong and congenial relationship at that time. This seemed to hold true up into the Middle Ages.

Between the time of the Greeks and the Middle Ages in Europe, an event of enormous importance occurred—the spread of Christianity. With it came radical changes in the theory and practice of human relationships which added new dimensions to the doctor-patient relationship. Among these were the Christian concepts of neighborliness and *agape* (a Greek word which literally means "love"), the emergence of the priest-doctor as the dominant figure in the healing arts, and the involvement of the State in the practice of medicine.

The Greek notion of *philia* was strengthened by the addition of the Christian concepts of neighborliness and *agape*, thus adding to the unique dimensions of the doctor-patient relationship. In the Christian context, the benevolent relationships between man are basically of two forms: neighborliness and friendship. Christians believed that anyone in need was their neighbor. Thus, a sick person in need of a cure was a neighbor of the doctor. To this was added the concept of *agape*, which is a form of love which renders help without expecting anything in return. These new ideas demanded that the doctor help the patient, first of all, because the patient was his neighbor, and second, because of the *agape* that existed between the two. It was considered to be the doctor's moral duty to preserve the body of the person in order to save the patient's soul.

Another change that occurred in the Middle Ages was that during the first half of the seventh century two different forms of doctors emerged: those who practiced monastic medicine, purely Christian, and those who were more secular in outlook. Medical treatment swiftly passed into the hands of the clergy, and priest-doctors became the dominant figures in the art of healing. In Italy in 529, Benedictine monasteries started to receive and care for the sick at Monte Cassino. In Spain, Pablo, who was bishop of Merida between 530 and 560, did not hesitate to take the knife to perform a Caesarean operation. In 580 the bishop of Merida founded a hospital, which was staffed by clergy.

As in ancient Greece, a patient in the days of medieval Christianity saw the doctor as an agent of God, and thus respected him highly, but did not expect more than the doctor could supply. Illness was viewed as an element of absolute necessity, a permanent possibility and part of man's nature. It was believed that there was a mysteriousness about certain diseases, which were thus incurable and the physician was powerless to deal with them. An Italian humorist said that it must be recognized that medicine is only useful and necessary in the case of curable illness.

The Church emphasized the preservation of the soul more than the healing of the body—the body was temporal, the soul eternal. Thus the body must be humiliated in order to save the soul. Early Church fathers preached the sinfulness of resorting to medicine as a cure for bodily ills and advocated instead trust in the intercession of saints—healing became a test of faith. For example, sick people who were considered to be possessed were seen by exorcists, a specific order of priests who expelled devils with a prescribed series of prayers invoking the saints. The disease was considered a supernatural visitation which required a supernatural intervention, and the Church ascribed this function to the saints, who followed in the footsteps of Christ. By calling on the saints, the doctor-priest participated in the attributes of God.

Around the turn of the thirteenth century, things took a sudden shift in medicine. Both society and the State exerted more and more influence over the relationship between doctor and patient. Frederick II decreed that a medical practitioner must have an official title. The decree also required the doctor to give free help to the poor, visit a sick man at least twice a day, and, if necessary, visit the patient every night as well. The doctor was not to charge extra for making house calls unless they were out-of-town, and even then limits were set on those fees. (The Greek doctor had kept out-of-town patients at his own house, where they were nursed by his assistants and slaves and kept under constant observation. By the Middle Ages this practice had declined considerably, although the doctor made the house calls required by law.)

The involvement of the State in the art of healing gave birth to the legal rationalization of the doctor-patient relationship, and it shifted from the Greek and Christian concepts of *philia* and *agape* to a contractual one. Then, for the first time in history, the prestige of the doctor declined. The doctor, before undertaking treatment, had to agree on his fee and also pay a sum of money as a deposit to the patient or his family as a security against malpractice. If the patient died, the doctor had no right to any fee, but could take back his deposit. Technical mistakes were punished in various ways: for a badly performed bloodletting, he was fined a specific amount of money. If a slave under treatment died, he had to provide another slave to the owner. If a freeman died, he must accept the arbitration of the family. It was no laughing matter to practice medicine in the Middle Ages.

So the doctor was well aware of the importance of maintaining a congenial relationship with the patient and knew that the most effective way to gain the patient's confidence and a personal rapport, establishing the bond of friendship, was through open communications. He made maximum use of his senses to establish this communication, and he made maximum use of his ears to listen to the patient. He did not have paramedicals to assist him; consequently, the patient's family played a great role in the treatment process.

The doctor in the Middle Ages was trained to look at each patient as an individual, as unique. It was believed that a good doctor-patient relationship depended on the historical and social circumstances under which they met, on the patient's personal attitude toward his own illness, toward medicine in general and his own doctor, and on the doctor's personal attitude toward the practice of his profession and toward this particular patient. In order to be effective, a doctor made himself fully aware both of the patient's biographical data and his motive for seeking medical treatment.

In the Middle Ages, the doctor and the patient enjoyed a more favorable relationship than they do now. Why? Was the patient more genuinely desirous of getting well? Was the patient inherently more reasonable and cooperative than the modern patient? As a rule, the sick man consults the doctor because he wants to get well, or stay well. However, even during the Middle Ages there were cases in which the dominant motive of the patient was for a diagnosis; they had an urgent need to know what was wrong. There were some who took refuge in illness. There were those who saw the doctor with fictitious symptoms. The patient did not always carry through with the course of treatment after finding out he was sick. The physician was well aware of the fact that even when the decision to consult a doctor seems autonomous and personal, it always contains a hidden reference to other people the patient always has in his mind—his wife, children, parents, and so on.

What strengthened the doctor-patient relationship was the type of medical practice. The doctor saw the patient as part of a family unit. He knew the family, and may have known the patient since he was born. He made house calls. He was there whenever the patient needed him, regardless of the type of illness or problem.

The success of the doctor-patient relationship in the Greek era and the Middle Ages seemed to have resulted from that philosophy of medical practice. Plato called medicine "the science of what pertains to the love of the body." The Greek and medieval physicians combined scientific knowledge, technical skills and love for the perfection of the human body to produce this enviable professional-client relationship.

How does the current doctor-patient relationship compare to those of early Greece and the Middle Ages? Not very well. In recent years there has been a marked deterioration in the doctor-patient relationship. Symptoms are patients quitting their doctors, the majority of citizens criticizing their physicians and medical care, patients not paying doctors' fees, patients turning to non-medical healers and fast-rising rates of malpractice suits confirm that the doctor and the patient do not enjoy a very congenial relationship. In fact, fifty percent of all patients have at one time or another quit their doctor because they were dissatisfied with him. An average of fifteen percent of all patients fail to pay their doctors' bills, and the main reason given for withholding payment is dissatisfaction with the physician.

At this point in time, the public view is that the medical profession is a clan or fraternity bound by internal solidarity to protect its erring members from public scrutiny or punitive action. The individual sees himself as a pebble which is helpless in attaining justice against the raging tides. The patient fears the doctor's loyalties will be first with his colleagues, and then with his patients. Consequently, the doctor and patient are not friends as they were in the Greek era and the Middle Ages.

Sixty-five percent of all patients criticize the way their doctors communicate with them. Patients complain that modern doctors lack human warmth—they might like the medical care, but not the way it is given. Seventy percent of adult patients express virulent dislike of the care they receive in hospitals; seventy percent approve of the use of nonmedical healers.

This breakdown in doctor-patient relations has been most noticeable in the increasing numbers of malpractice suits. Malpractice suits often are brought not because of any actual physical damage done, but rather as a reflection of the frustrated patient's dissatisfaction with their doctor. The patient feels that nobody gives a darn about him while the doctor feels that the patient is uncooperative and has unreasonable expectations. Indeed, the doctor seems to hold the patient entirely responsible—the doctor's concept of the situation excludes the practitioner from bearing any responsibility for the deterioration of the doctor-patient relationship.

Yet, the public image of the medical doctor is the most important factor which affects the doctor-patient relationship. The public sees the doctor as a person who has the best job, the most prestige, power and money. Inevitably, this exposes the physician to popular envy and intense criticism. The patient, in voicing his unfavorable sentiments against the doctor, is merely expressing the societal norm.

Television portrays an image of the medical practitioner and his profession which is far too idealistic to be realistic. The doctor is shown as a self-sacrificing individual who is not bothered in the least about remuneration. He is cool, calm and congenial and sees patients as though he has all the time in the world. He is shown having meals with the patient and his family. He smiles and even cracks a few jokes to cheer up the patient. In some cases, the doctor travels miles to meet and explain to the parents of a sick child the possible outcomes of a medical procedure. And the result of this is that the average patient, on entering the doctor's office or hospital, may expect his doctor to be no less than the doctor he saw on television.

The news media and the entertainment industry have over-sold the public about the self-sacrificing humanity of physicians and the unlimited success of medical science—some people really do believe that the "Six Million Dollar Man" was a real patient. Having seen the unlimited power of medical science on television, the patient blames the doctor for not making him well. The patient demonstrates animistic-magical thinking by imagining the doctor to be a magician who can cure all diseases. Contrary to the concept held by patients of ancient Greece and the Middle Ages, the modern patient believes the doctor himself is omnipotent. Some patients think of their doctor as the magical messenger of death or life, an attribute usually ascribed only to gods.

Eastern and Western medicine provide startling contrasts. The common man in China will accept science if it is disguised as magic, whereas the common man in America will accept magic if it is disguised as science. Thus the American patient, in the name of science, calls upon the magical power of the medical profession through its practitioners.

2

MD DOES NOT STAND FOR MEDICAL DEITY

In the vast majority of interviews we conducted, the phrase "doctors are gods" was used. Sometimes this was said in jest, sometimes just in passing. Sometimes the remark was made with concern, and sometimes it was said with contempt.

While this remark was made about physicians, we saw it as indicative of how our culture views medicine as a whole. Then there are the particular problems that the concept of the doctor as a god has created, from creating an unfair burden on doctors to clean up the mess many patients have made of their bodies and their lives, to creating a system where physician arrogance is not only tolerated, it is expected.

I think when you look at the health-care industry as a whole, the real problem isn't that we deal with life and death. That's not what makes it difficult. What makes it difficult is that the system has created these godlike creatures who in reality are only human. But it fails to recognize them as such and gives them license to behave as though they are God. It's crazy. That's where the real problem in health care lies.

Doctors and mankind are products of their culture, a culture that exerts a most significant influence in shaping ideas about sickness and health among people. One researcher studied hospitalized patients from four ethnic groups: Jewish, Italian, Irish and "Old Americans." It was observed that the Jewish and the Italians exaggerated their pain; the Irish were stoical and able to take a lot of pain, and that "Old Americans" were more objective about pain. Both the Italians and the Jewish were found to be quite uninhibited in the expression of pain. They felt free to groan, cry and moan. A doctor's lack of understanding of the culture of his patient may make him label the patient as difficult or unreasonable and is obviously going to affect the professional-client relationship.

Language has a marked impact on doctor-patient relationships. The physician and the patient who cannot communicate in the same language feel uneasy with each other. Religion, too, is a powerful influence. The doctor who overlooks the patient's religious world may invite problems and may even find himself misinterpreting the patient's comments. Many religious people see disease as proof of God's displeasure over their sins. Socioeconomic factors influence the doctor-patient relationship, as well. Social class not only dictates the activities of the patient, but also influences the way the health-care providers act toward the patient. Ability to pay is directly related to social class. It will influence how one is treated if one seeks free-clinic care, chiropractic and naturopathic cures, the moderately priced general practitioner or the high-priced specialist.

Specialization has brought poor communication. In contrast to the good old days when the family doctor was a jack-of-all-trades, the sick person today receives medical care from a team of physicians. The complexity of modern medical techniques may have brought quality of service; however, it has made it virtually impossible for the patient to establish a meaningful relationship with his physician. The specialist is too busy to take the time to know the patient personally. Each specialist sees illness not as a human problem but as a scientific problem. He tends to treat an illness rather than a human being. He reads the signs and symptoms off medical gadgets instead of studying the patient as a person. He knows more about the scientific world than the human world.

Doctors are gods—or are they? Does anyone really believe that? And yet, physicians and the medicine they practice have been elevated to a sacred place in our culture. Cloaked in science, distanced by technology, the separation between physicians and lay people, between those blessed with the power to heal and those in need of healing, seems to have widened in the last generation. Only to those working in the health-care industry, the mystery isn't so real, or the separation so distinct. Maybe it's time to rethink our expectations of medicine and the people who practice it. After all, we're only mortal human beings playing in the realm of immortality.

"Doctors are gods?" No. I think doctors are kings. Ask any hospital employee. Any of them, from the administrator down to the kitchen staff. Doctors are kings. Worse yet, child-kings. Not all of them, but some of them can throw a temper tantrum that makes you want to bend them over your knee and wail the daylights out of them. Those definitely consider themselves kings. "How dare you challenge my authority? I'm the doctor. Off with her head!" I learned early to determine which one had the sharpest knife with which to decapitate me.

Doctors are humans. The medical profession is in a position where they can do no wrong, so they scream like hell when you tell them that they screwed up. They say, "How do you know? You're not a doctor."

It's a strange thing. If you go into a doctor's office and he says, "Take off all your clothes and stand in the corner," you'll do it without question. As time goes on, the doctor comes to believe he is a god.

Many patients just dive into the system and let it carry them wherever. They're on a raft and in the surf and just go where the flow is.

There's a lot of ignorance seen in the way people have a set idea on what medicine should do, what they think should happen when they walk through the doors. And then, they don't always like what they get. They want this definite science which says "Yes, this is the problem. This is the treatment. Guaranteed. Here. Now go home and be well."

A broken bone is easy. You go in, you take an x-ray, stick a cast on it, and you're out the door. But most medicine isn't clear, cut-and-dried. You don't always know how to diagnose what you can't see. Diagnosis and treatment go by other things, too, such as the patient's history. It's often a guessing game and people don't always like that. They want to know exactly what's going on. Immediately. Without the possibility of error.

Before this industrial age of medicine, and especially in the last couple of generations, everybody accepted and knew that they were going to die. Mortality was very prominent—and evident. Longevity meant thirty or forty years. If you lived up into your sixties or seventies, you were the exception. It seems to me that as longevity has increased, our fear of death has increased as well. As medicine gets better and better and better at prolonging life, people are looking towards it to prevent them from ever having to die, to keep them from what is inevitable.

I think society now, not just medicine per se, but everything in our culture, is geared toward "We're determined to keep you alive longer. We're going to make you better, new and improved. The longer you live, the better you'll live and the happier you'll be." As if the only measure of our life is duration.

When someone thirty finds out they have cancer, it's, "Oh, my God! Do something! Change something! Make something different!" A hundred years ago, if someone were to die at thirty, it wasn't uncommon. Today, our society is so frightened of death that it's almost thought of as an unnatural part of the life process, and medicine is expected to be the intervention there that changes that. People are saying, "Do something, you have the power." Well, we don't have the power at all to prevent death.

People don't want to be sick—at all. I'm not saying it's pleasant, but it is a part of our human makeup, to be ill and to die. That just happens. People just don't seem to be comfortable with that. They want the medicines to cure everything. They want the diagnosis accurate and complete. They want tons of money poured into research.

An eighty year old, comatose patient will be admitted to the hospital, and we hear their family say, "Do everything for them. We want to make them a full cardiopulmonary resuscitation." I'm thinking, "You're kidding. They're eighty." The family will insist. "Do open-heart surgery on them. Replace all the valves. You might be able to get that heart to last ten more years." I think medicine is being asked to do, forced to do, what it is not intended to do.

I don't care what any doctor, or any patient, or especially any lawyer says, doctors are not gods. They're human beings just like you and me, and as such, they're going to make an occasional mistake. To hold them to a divine standard is preposterous. It's true, they've got a lot more head knowledge than anybody else when it comes to the workings of the human body, but in spite of all those years of education, they don't have a supernatural ability to diagnose and treat disease. What they are able to do is make an educated guess. And that's all they're doing—guessing.

When a doctor is trying to diagnose a patient, they are simply "ruling out" everything that it could not be. Not compiling a list of symptoms and saying, "Oh, it's obviously this." They rule out by saying, "OK, it's not this, and it's not this and it's not this." Some of it is pretty exact, some isn't. With a bladder infection, you do urine test and discover high white cells and a few other indicators, and then you can say, "Yeah, that's a bladder infection." Can you always, one hundred percent, rule out that it isn't coming from the kidney? Not always. So before you say it's a bladder infection, you have to rule out that it's not the kidneys. Do you understand the concept? A doctor figures out what the ailment is by determining what it is not, and then says, "This is my best guess." Fortunately, he's been trained thoroughly and is generally good at guessing.

Sometimes he rules out by prescribing a method or a medicine for treatment. Maybe it doesn't alleviate the symptoms. Maybe he was wrong in his diagnosis. That doesn't make him a bad doctor. That's how the system works. So he takes another guess, and tries something else. He'll continue this until he finally hits the right treatment.

S ome patients will even tell the doctor what they want done, and the doctor will be pushed into a corner by the patient and feel they have to do it. So many patients are willing to just be mad at the doctors and blame them for diagnosing something wrong. Most of the time, medicine is not an exact science. Yet that's when people show up and say, "You're going to tell me exactly what's wrong with my arm, why I've got pain in it. You're going to x-ray it. Even if nothing shows up on x-ray, you're going to tell me exactly what's wrong and you're going to give me medicine, and you're to make it better."

I nsurance companies will win well over half the cases that go to trial. Right now it's about seventy percent, so seven out of ten malpractice cases—and they're usually pretty good malpractice cases—will be lost by the patient at trial. Juries have a hard time, and I think it's true for the general public too, but juries have a hard time finding malpractice against a doctor. It's like a doctor is absolute. He can do no wrong. He went to medical school, therefore, he's supposed to be infallible.

M ost people don't understand that when a malpractice insurance company settles a case on behalf of a doctor, they have to do it with the written approval of the doctor. You better know on those cases, for sure, the doctor was dead, flat wrong, or he would have never signed an authorization.

I f a doctor does make a mistake, a pharmacist has to get on the phone to him and tell him. I think there's always some animosity involved. It's an ego thing, I suppose. We're not trying to second guess the doctor, but that's our job, that's what I went to school for six years to learn.

If the physician has ordered the wrong drug and refuses to change it, I handle it simply. I just refuse to fill the order. Of course, that's a very difficult thing for me to do, because if you're too strong, you can get blackballed by the physicians, and that's the end of your business. So you have to be very tactful in how you let a doctor know he's made a mistake. In the majority of the cases, I think the physician appreciates what I'm saying, but there's always a bit of animosity.

Hospital administrators' disputes with physicians will usually end with the administrator getting fired or quitting. The doctor brings money to the hospital, the administrator doesn't. It's always easier to find another manager because the physician can take his patients down the road to another facility. That's why a hospital administrator is defined as a person who has just taken a job and is looking for another. The average length of employment of administrators in over 6,000 hospitals is slightly over one year. Doctors usually stay until they retire. What does that tell you?

When questioned about doctors of suspect character, hospital managers have found that the only safe answer is, "He or she is a good doctor." But they will never tell you that they would only refer their enemies to them.

There's a greater diversity of people that are physicians these days. Some are extremely good and extremely compassionate human beings. They're people who can sit down and talk about something other than the stock market. You know, just sit down and have a normal conversation, have the same goals, have the same problems, talk to you on an equal basis. That said, I've been fifteen years in the health-care field and I don't have a physician that I can call a friend. They do not associate with non-physicians. It's very much a caste system.

There is something in their training, in their makeup, that

makes them unapproachable, that makes them not fit into what we consider normal. I've been told that it's because they have to play God, because they're told that their decision is unquestioned. I don't know how healthy that is, I've always thought that. I mean, the best doctors that I've ever met are those that are willing to ask questions. And that's been my philosophy, professionally and personally. My god, you're just being stupid if you don't know something and won't ask. And they don't ask.

I t must be something in their training, in their Philosophy 101 that they take. We call it Asshole 101.

A s the hospital food service manager, what really pisses me off is these doctors that feel they should never have to pay for their food. As if they can't afford it! They come into the cafeteria, fill up a tray and head for the conference room. If the cashier tries to ring it up, they tell them that they're working at a committee meeting and are entitled to a free lunch. They can be quite intimidating. Well, somebody has to pay for it, so the hospital ends up passing on the cost to the patients.

The worst offender is an old dermatologist. He's constantly complaining because he doesn't like our breakfasts. He wants a special short-order cook on staff just for him. When I mentioned it to another doctor, one who actually pays for his meals, he laughed and said, "Don't worry about it. He's so cheap he even has meters in the parking lot of his medical building." I know it's a joke, but it wouldn't surprise me.

I think a perfect story is something that happened today. We had a patient that needed lab work drawn. She was originally scheduled for surgery last month. Came in for all the pre-op work and something wasn't normal, so the doctor canceled the surgery. Now she's scheduled for surgery Monday and she came in again today. We still had the blood work from a month before but needed new labs done. She refused and just had a cow about it.

It's very interesting because patients sometimes will reflect the same personality as the doctor. I think it's amazing. You know, like dogs will look like their owners. Same sort of schizophrenic behavior with these two.

I took it upon myself to call the doctor's office to inform him that this patient refused, that blood work will not be on the chart and available for Monday's surgery. I get the phone call back from the doctor and he just reams me a new asshole. He said that the patient didn't change, nothing had changed, and we were gouging and we were stupid and all this other stuff. I told him on a real factual basis why we had to do it. It's required by the ABB standards, the FDA, the state of California, JCAHO. And he said, "Well those are all a bunch of fucking standards."

That is a physician's attitude: Don't tell me immutable facts. If I say so, it doesn't matter. It's not important. And that's what we have to deal with, all of us have had to deal with it.

A good physician may have objected but asked, "Why is that?" Then I could have spoken to them in intelligent, adult terms. Not gone down to the grade-school level, throwing four letter words out.

I wonder how doctors treat people outside the hospital? If one went down to the hardware store and engaged in a conversation with the clerk behind the counter and said, "Well, I want an eight-thirty-seconds drill that looks like this," and the clerk said, "I'm sorry, they don't make one of those." Would a doctor pound his fist and scream and call the clerk names? I really wonder. I'd be fascinated to know.

One radiologist, he was a billy goat, he was just a good old boy. I remember one case where they were doing a hystero-salpingiogram—fallopian tubes. You have to prep the area with Betadine before you go into a woman's private parts, and he was singing "Rub-a-dub-dub, three men in a tub," as he was prepping her.

Same character told one overweight lady as she was being laid down on a table to have a barium enema, "Hey, you win first prize at the county fair."

He was chairman of the department for a while.

I called him the Prussian. He was a surgeon whose unsuccessful practice made him work as a general practitioner. That meant a surgical cure for everything. He was an older man who developed a major practice. In the days before Medicare restrictions he would admit ten new patients a day to the hospital. He was a workaholic who commanded respect from his elderly patients because of the force of his personality. He was tall, muscular and pedantic. Organized to a fault, he dominated the scene. He was never challenged professionally on his practice of medicine, his case management never was carefully scrutinized. Other physicians were afraid of him because he kept records of their mistakes—a vigorous offense was the best defense for Joe. Joe wasn't an incompetent physician, his problem was that he needed to be acknowledged and respected beyond normal needs.

My first combat with him occurred my first day at work as the new administrator. As soon as my car stopped in the parking lot, a nurse ran up to me shouting that Dr. Joe wanted me in surgery immediately because of an emergency. I quickly went to the surgical suite and asked the supervising nurse what the problem was. She just smiled and suggested that I change into surgical clothes and see for myself, so I quickly dressed in mask and gown.

"Come in!" he ordered. I entered the operating room. It was unbearably hot. The operating lights focused heat on an open abdomen. Dr. Joe was moving things around while shouting at a nurse to wipe his brow. He stopped for a second, stared at me and said, "The air-conditioning in this room doesn't work, hasn't worked for a long time, and if any of my sweat causes an infection in this patient, it will personally be your fault. Now get your ass out of here and fix the problem."

What a way to start a day! I was happy to change into my street clothes and get out of the department of surgery. Rather than going to my office, I went directly to the hospital engineer's office. When I explained the problem to the engineer he responded in anger, "Tell the old fart to keep his hands off of the thermostat!" Apparently Dr. Joe had the habit of going into surgery the night before his cases and turning up the thermostat to maximum air conditioning. When he began operating at 7:30 a.m. the next day, the air conditioning units on the roof were close to icing over. Soon the units would stop because the condenser would be completely iced up. No air would move into the operating room. The engineer had explained the problem repeatedly to Dr. Joe, who was totally deaf on the matter.

I solved the problem quickly. Dr. Joe would never understand that his manipulation of the thermostat was the problem. I instructed the engineer to disconnect the existing thermostat and to install a new one in an obscure location in the room. It worked! Dr. Joe would still come in the night before surgery and fiddle with the thermostat so that the operating room would be cold. He never knew that he had been tricked.

Joe was in control of his medical practice. His patients were elderly or poor and they would comply faithfully with his orders. They were his fans, even though the poor souls didn't realize the enormous overutilization of services ordered by their doctor. And Joe really knew how to maximize his practice's income. He put an x-ray unit into his office and was able to barely meet the licensing requirements for the unit, but he did. Every patient was given a full set of x-rays on every occasion. Joe couldn't interpret the films, so he sent them to the hospital's radiologist for reading. I learned that Joe paid only twenty percent for this service and billed the insurance company or the patient the full amount. He quickly paid for the purchase of the x-ray machine which became a steady source of unchallenged income.

Joe's appetite was so whetted by the x-ray profits that he decided to establish a clinical laboratory in his office. He contacted a major reference laboratory who had no objections of equipping and staffing such an operation—both would earn enormous profits if enough patients were involved. The clinical laboratory was legal and was certified by state inspectors. What was wrong was the overutilization of that service. To increase the profits, Dr. Joe would order lab work to be performed "stat," which meant premium reimbursement. Joe also served as the "house doctor" for convalescent hospitals and nursing homes in the area. He may have had as many as 500 patients in his practice from this source. Most of these patients were confused and without interested family members and Joe made it a practice to order, at least monthly, a panel of eighteen laboratory tests on every patient. It was rumored that most of the specimens were never tested, but only given the "sink test." This meant that the blood specimen was poured down the sink without examination and an estimated result was prepared.

Panel tests are usually performed by one machine that has computerized results. Joe's laboratory performed each test on an individual basis. Charging on an itemized basis permitted Joe to increase the profits to five times greater. Between the x-ray and the laboratory, he was becoming a very wealthy man.

Then Joe did a self-diagnosis of some extremely rare, textbook heart disease and began treating himself. He made it worse by having two sets of consultants who were not aware of the other's existence. Two sets of consultants, each prescribing different medications, in combination with his own self-prescribed medications caused real problems.

Joe was in a medication stupor while driving his car far above the speed limit on a major interstate highway. Even though his car was totalled, he didn't have any serious injuries. It was a miracle. After examination at another hospital's emergency room, he was released. About six in the evening, I was notified of his admission on the second floor. One of his personal consultants wanted him to have an overnight observation.

I went into Joe's room to find him pacing like a caged animal. He was extremely distressed and wanted to talk about very private things in his life. He shared with me his personal problems and history. As a young physician he became addicted to drugs and temporarily lost his license to practice medicine. He felt he was a horrible father and husband.

I suggested that he shouldn't confess to me, it wasn't appropriate, but he kept right on talking. He said I was the best available listener at that moment, and he needed to talk. He told of his marital indiscretions and that he was currently having a torrid affair with one of the young married nurses on duty at that time.

In between his pacing and crying, he would sit quietly staring at the ceiling. Four hours later I went home. Joe was resting comfortably and in no apparent distress.

It seemed that I was no sooner asleep when the telephone next to my bed rang. The supervising nurse called to tell me that Dr. Joe had signed out against medical advice and had checked himself into a local hotel. Several hours later, the hospital telephoned again. Dr. Joe was dead on arrival in the emergency room. His mistress, a married nurse, had given him the final treatment for his heart. He died. End of story.

I think the most deceitful physician that I crossed paths with was a cardiologist.

He was a man of great potential and charisma. He was born in a progressive foreign country, and he grew up in wealth and privilege. He was the top graduate of his medical school and had a brilliant scientific future. His life-style far exceeded his countrymen but it wasn't enough, so this doctor packed his papers, credentials, dancing shoes and headed for the States.

He was tall, dark, muscular and handsome. He also brought along with him a wealthy, attractive wife. What a beautiful couple. The physicians in our community were impressed. There were no signs of greed or character flaws. Doors opened quickly. All of the cardiologists in the city wanted him to join their practices. The hospital's credentials committee was impressed. Every report on him was glowing.

In order to become a member of the hospital's medical staff, he was required to make a personal appearance before some of the staff committees. He really put on a show. We had a real need for more cardiologists in our community; our emergency room always needed more heart specialists on call. He was a gift from above.

His private practice began strongly, and it was no time before he was busy all of the time. In contrast to her cool, calm and collected husband, his wife was volatile and fiery. Their marriage appeared to be sound and full of love. In fact, they were a charming couple.

He became very flamboyant in soliciting friends. He had his favorite restaurant where he was king. The maitre d' would escort him and his guest to the best table with a flourish. His favorite cocktail would be delivered without being ordered. Nothing was too good for him and he showered the hospital community with social favors.

The various medical staff committees at the hospital who were charged with assuring quality health care found no criticism in his treatment of patients. He did everything right, and quickly moved up the medical staff organization ladder. It was no time before some other doctors suggested that he become the paid director of the Cardiac Intensive Care Unit. Soon there were suggestions that he develop a cardiac rehabilitation program at the hospital.

The operating room nurses loved him. He was charming and gracious. He never lost his temper or made unreasonable demands. He was always busy implanting pacemakers. Normally a thoracic surgeon makes the cut into the chest, but he did that task faster and better than other staff doctors.

A year went by and he was well on his way to a tremendous practice. There was an occasional storm cloud when another cardiologist would question the advisability of a permanent pacemaker. These concerns were dismissed without investigation by other physicians as being motivated by jealousy. Meanwhile the wife had developed a reputation of being a yeller and screamer, a woman with chronic PMS, so rumors of his extra-marital affairs were expected.

One day, the hospital staff was shocked to learn that one of the hospital nurses had died of a drug overdose. She was young, blonde and very attractive. One would have never suspected she had a problem. Her performance and demeanor at the hospital was always professional. Then a dark secret became gossip. One of the supervising nurses mentioned that the dead nurse had been having an affair with the doctor, and that he had attempted to break it off. The police investigation did not reveal any additional information, other than she had died of an accidental overdose of drugs.

So the incident was soon forgotten. But several months later there was another employee death. Another young, attractive girl, a telephone operator, had committed suicide and had left a note saying that the father of her unborn child refused to help her. Gossip had it that this doctor was her lover. Like the other girl, nothing ever came of the investigation of her death.

It wasn't long before he became the topic of whispered conversations. The substance of the comments was that he would court the lady in grand style and then would remove any resistance with the help of a little medication. He always left the scene as quickly as he arrived. It's said that one day after seeing his last patient in the office, he opened a package that had been delivered earlier in the afternoon. Bloodcurdling screams could be heard in the building. When he lifted the lid to the box, he found a rattlesnake inside.

Was it from his wife, a girlfriend, or a patient? Nobody knows. He just left town. Word was he had returned to his native land.

H e was a collector of wives and mistresses. His sexual conquests of female hospital employees were legendary, but instead of being criticized for this behavior, he was admired by many as being a harmless Don Juan.

I remember his third wife as a very attractive woman—she should have been. He'd had his plastic surgery friends reconstruct every important part of her anatomy. He was so proud of the sex machine he had created, he would joyfully offer her services to any interested male.

He was the busiest physician at the hospital—on any given day he was treating thirty percent of the patients, with another thirty percent having been referred to surgical specialists. It was the custom that the specialist would ask the referring doctor to assist in routine cases, in that way the specialist would continue to get referrals.

To his patients he was a god. He delivered babies, practiced pediatrics, did most of the internal medicine and had a great bedside manner. His main surgical procedure was the hysterectomy, and he always had an influential surgeon or family practitioner assisting him—he knew how to circle the wagons for protection. He ran his own kingdom. He was never sued because he only admitted patients first seen in his office—where he could build rapport and trust. He always worked alone in his office, so there was no opportunity for his patients to compare him with another physician. Responsible physicians refused to be on the hospital medical staff with him, and preferred to travel to the neighboring city's hospital rather than be associated with him.

This guy sounds like he was just a successful entrepreneur—maybe his testicles were a little overactive? *Wrong.* He was a sex addict who used his confidential position to identify potential sexual partners.

If there was a woman who sparked his sexual interest, he would work every angle to get her to be examined by a psychiatric consultant in gynecology. What the lady wouldn't know is that the consulting physician had a unique interest—sexual dysfunction. This consultant readily established rapport with the patient, who would confess her secrets and inner feelings, many of which had been long repressed. After several visits, the patient would be referred back to our friend, who by then would have been provided with a written consultation report of the specialist's examination. He would then know what buttons to push to get the lady flat on her back—or any other position of lust.

There's nothing illegal about physicians sharing information. It was good medical practice to send the referring physician a detailed report so the patient's medical record would be complete. But it was immoral to use such confidential information for personal gain.

This doctor is still flourishing. He married another young woman who had been his mistress during his last marriage. She is scheduled for a tummy tuck and a breast augmentation. Another perfect sex machine is being created to share with friends, enemies and strangers.

Physicians tend to have larger egos than the general public, and some of them do not want to be told that they could do something wrong. It's just not within their conception of themselves. There's even a degree of paranoia about it.

Interestingly, people who go to medical school, prior to going

to medical school, are one standard deviation significantly more
paranoid than the general public to start with. I think the medical
education system that we have in this country and Canada tends
to exacerbate that. It's much more cutthroat than the rest of the
world.

There have been studies that indicate that the personalities of
physicians tend to be more problematical than the general public.
There is a large substance abuse problem within the profession.
Although the general public would probably think the contrary,
people who select to go into medicine often have more problems.

There is no curriculum for personal growth in medical
schools. Training physician missionaries for society has
never existed.

The educational process destroys the natural empathy of the
medical student. The process is like boot camp, but worse. Fear,
intimidation, physical and mental exhaustion are the educators
and the modifiers of values.

I've witnessed, over the years, the high turnover of personnel
many doctors have. Not all doctors—I don't want to classify
them all like that—but there's a percentage of them out there
that are so egotistical and arrogant that people won't stay with
them. I know it's true, because everyone who works for these doctors agrees with me, except for the office manager, and she's usually the doctor's wife.

The doctors that still have the power and still have the most
arrogant attitudes are the ones that bring patients into the
hospital. Those are basically the cardiologists, any type of surgeon, and internal medicine guys. Those three and, to a much
lesser extent because there are not that many of them, general
practitioners or family practitioners. Those are the ones that actually bring revenue into the hospital.

But their power is waning as they become wrapped up in these
Health Maintenance Organization and Preferred Provider Orga-

nization and managed care contracts. They're being forced to go into them to get their patients and their money. All of that's changing, their arrogance, their thoughtlessness is going away.

T here was a time that if a doctor was treating you like shit there was nothing you could do. But nowadays if you have a grievance of that sort of thing, there's a means of going about it. There's been several times at our facility that the administrators have gone to doctors and said, "Listen, you can't treat these people like this. This person is threatening to quit and sue us." These doctors aren't stupid. They don't want to be hassled. They'll generally lay off.

S cript writers for television and motion pictures perpetuate the image of the all powerful physician who expertly does anything and everything. I think the best example is Dr. Marcus Welby. Dr. Welby was omnipotent. He did everything that in the real world would be performed only by a dozen other specialists.

When Dr. Welby entered the hospital he walked on water. This kindly family doctor whose training was limited to four years of medical school and one year of rotating internship had all of the skills of every highly trained medical and surgical specialist. Board-certified specialists are trained for an additional two to eight years after completion of an internship. That means dear old Dr. Welby had the specialty skills requiring at least forty years of advanced education. If he had taken all that training, he would have been eligible for Medicare benefits before starting his practice of medicine.

Dr. Marcus Welby is a god, at least in the mind of script writers and millions of television viewers. How disappointed they must be when in real life they discover that there "ain't no Welby" to give them the medical care they want.

P eople think that we know more than we do. It's true that it can be a real disappointment. Sometimes that grows because a lot of doctors forget to be humble and sort of feed into that thought that "we know everything." We don't. There's a lot we don't know.

We disappoint people because they think we know more than we do about how the body functions and about how to fix it.

I think a lot of it now is people's expectations of medical care. They have been programmed to always expect more. Everything is magnified in their thinking. Now it's not just a cold, it's pneumonia. It's not a sore throat, it's strep. It's not indigestion, it's a myocardial infarction. It's not the flu, it's cancer.

Maybe if we got back to a more realistic view of what medicine can do, that it can't cure everything, it can't take away all our pain, maybe then we'd get away from suing anybody and everybody who fails doing those things. That alone would bring down the costs.

It's in our values also, how we've changed from the fifties to the sixties. There was an end in some respects of self-responsibility. I'm responsible for what I do, and I bring my children up to think that way, too. Then our system shifted to where it was everybody else's responsibility. We shifted that responsibility outside of the home and outside of ourselves. I'm a Mid-westerner and that's the value system I grew up with. But there are a lot of people out there today who want to allow the government to be responsible or other people to be responsible, but then if something goes wrong, those others ought to pay.

I feel strongly that medicine and health care are not a total science. There's still an art involved with it. We do a lot for ourselves by learning about our health care and taking care of ourselves that doctors can't be responsible for.

Part of that, doctors did themselves. Remember the god era? "Don't worry your little head about this, I'll take care of it. You don't have to know anything about it."

Because I've been in the profession for a while, I see that my role is simply to be a servant and to help people. That's why I've been given this profession. It's not just to allow me to increase my income. I have to remind myself of that every time I finish an exam.

T hings are changing. The guys that would throw stuff and demean you and do all kinds of little tricks to screw you up are disappearing. I don't know whether it's because they're just a different type of people going into medicine these days, or if it's because they've just gotten the snot beat out of them during their residency. The younger docs are actually fun to work with. They're nice guys or ladies for the most part, more down-to-earth. They don't have this arrogant "the doctor is here and everybody else is down the nose" attitude.

I think that's going to happen all the more as they're no longer making $500,000 or $850,000 a year. They're making $150,000 or $200,000 a year. It's still a lot more than technologists and nurses make, but it's not as big of a gap as it used to be.

Also, they're treated by hospital administration and by department administrators the same way as everybody else is because, in a lot of hospitals, they're just employees, too.

O ur country gave doctors all kinds of protection. Our laws have allowed all that freedom. Now, I think we're trying to take some of that back. I support it. It's ridiculous that we don't do more in terms of monitoring the practitioners—physicians, nurses or whoever. But it's namely the physicians who have had way too much freedom, like the spoiled child, and the whole thing stinks. But I don't think it's going to change without having continuous pressure from the public.

W hy do people believe that doctors are capable of making completely accurate diagnoses and infallible decisions about therapies for various diseases? Why do juries give outlandish judgments based on the principle of medical infallibility, and therefore a physician must pay exceedingly if a patient suffers an injury in the course of medical treatment. The answer is obvious. Doctors are gods and gods do not make mistakes.

W hen a physician refuses to acknowledge his own limitations, the ones that eventually lead to social unhappiness and medical disaster, he's playing God.

Physicians come from the same general population as any other profession. Statistically, they have a similar number of drug-impaired members. They have a similar incidence of psychiatric problems. And their hormones rage at the same varying levels. Health care has the same wide range of moral and ethical values and problems that are found in the general population. Our dissatisfaction begins with an unwillingness to accept less than perfection in professions that can affect us directly. Do we expect more from doctors than we do other professions? You bet we do. Do we have a right to expect more? You bet we do!

Doctors get trained on old sick people in the hospital. Then they graduate and start a private practice totally unprepared for patients who are hypochondriacs, psychologically immature and uneducated regarding their own bodies. The real challenge to a new doctor is not the sick patients, but the healthy ones who only need a swift kick in the rear-end.

A license to practice medicine is a privilege earned as a result of intensive study and abdication of the rights of leisure. Becoming a physician requires intelligence and extreme discipline. Basic training in the Marines is far easier than the year of hell of being a medical intern. Basic training is only eight to sixteen weeks with fairly regular hours for sleep. The year of being an intern is a physical and emotional marathon that runs 24 hours a day. Doing specialty training is even more demanding. Exhaustion can led to permanent personality changes.

Being a physician awards a privilege to hear a patient's innermost thoughts and fears, to see a person naked, to poke into every body orifice, to commit mayhem by sticking with needles, to cut a patient open and to poison with dangerous drugs. Patients and relatives thank and pay physicians for performing all of the above indignities, which if a stranger did it by force would result in a police complaint. People go to jail for what doctors do with consent.

M edical schools do not select humanitarians. They prefer nerds because nerds are usually high achievers. The fact that nerds tend to be socially inept is not a disqualification. Medical schools look for the 4.0 grade point student. If they have no obvious physical or psychological handicaps, a nerd can pass the selection process rather easily.

T he nature of medical school doesn't create human beings. Therefore, medical students tend to be more academic and fiercely competitive. The result is technical skills without an intuitive nature.

A nesthesiologists have known for a long time a fact that surgeons to this day refuse to recognize. Even under anesthesia, the patient is subconsciously aware of what is going on. When the surgeon says, "this poor bastard is not going to make it," the patient surely will lose the will to survive.

S ome doctors just have the magic. They don't require lots of testing or consultations. They can sense what is wrong. Maybe it's because they know how to take and understand the patient's medical history. They rely equally on what the patient says as well as the lab reports.

I remember early in my training waiting to start an exploratory surgery with a team of other young doctors. While waiting in the surgeons' lounge, this old-timer stopped in for a cup of coffee and a bran muffin. We were discussing the impending surgery while he quietly listened. Shortly, he offered his opinion of the patient's problem. We couldn't laugh at the old guy. That would have been rude. But were we ever surprised to learn when we opened the patient up that the old-timer was right.

I would be hesitant of going into a teaching hospital unless I identified who it was that was going to do a surgical procedure on me. Also it's common knowledge that you want to avoid going into the hospital in July because July 1st is when the new interns

start. They're just overwhelmed and the quality of care you're going to get at that point is not as good as a month or preferably two
or three months later.

Mortality rates of teaching hospitals are still frightening.
When a new group of interns starts, the death rate and
complication rate is at it highest level for the year. Towards the
end of the internship, patients have a better chance of survival.
This is probably the origin for "doctors bury their mistakes."

My first night as an intern in a hospital was a nightmare for
me. It must have been worse for my patients. I was assigned to a forty-bed pediatrics ward. I started with twenty-two
patients and had ten admissions. I was on duty for 36 hours
straight. That meant that I was on my feet almost the entire time.
I didn't even have time to pee. On that service was a senior resident and a second-year resident. Theoretically, they were available for consultation. Quickly I learned that to ask questions of
them would only bring abuse and humiliation. I wanted to quit
being a doctor that night. The misgivings I had for my career
choice staggered me.

Fortunately a couple of years ago the marathon 36-to-48-hour
assignments for interns ended with a revolt of the interns. Working with various professional societies like the American Medical
Association brought on reform of working hours and tradition.
The macho pride of having survived the boot camp of medical
hell was replaced by reason. No longer did the "I survived the
ordeal and so must you," prevail. Now interns and residents are
limited to 12-hour shifts.

The damage done by age-old practices of training doctors is
still with us. Ninety percent of practicing physicians still bear the
scars of the brutality of the training experience.

Morning report destroyed what little humanism remained. I
had to have all of the answers at the tip of my tongue. The
patient lost his personal identity. He ceased to have a name, but

only a diagnosis. The patient became the "gall bladder in room five," not a total person in need of healing and comfort. To survive the shift, all patients had to become diagnoses and not personalities. Internship was the turning point in not being human, but only a technocrat.

The medical students who fail to overachieve in academics, become the dropouts of medicine—the general practice doctors, the pathologists, the radiologists and the psychiatrists. A lot of other physicians think the shrinks really shouldn't be called doctors. Although these types of doctors have less respect from within the profession, they tend to be more humanistic.

There is a real difference between osteopathic physicians and medical doctors. The educational curriculum for both types is similar, although the osteopaths conceptually believe that the spine and manipulative techniques have curative powers in addition to standard medical treatments. Doctors of osteopathy have better rapport with their patients than MDs do, probably because they have something to prove for not being selected by "MD" medical schools. That is a fact of life. Good students not selected by MD medical schools have no choice but to apply for "DO" medical schools. DOs always seem to have something to prove for their rejection. Lacking professional prestige, they strive to be superior in the only way they can—by being good listeners.

There's a certain segment that thinks modern medicine will solve all their problems and allow them to be a hundred and never be sick. That's unrealistic. Deep down inside, we all know it. Some people want to address every social ill, throw money at it and make it go away. It doesn't work. You can't solve death. We're all going to die. Expecting somebody, someplace, to intervene and keep us alive forever is unrealistic.

Until we've conquered mortality, the American people will not be satisfied with their health care. I wonder if anyone will hear this? Guess what—we've set an impossible standard of care. It's never going to happen. We're all going to die. Everyone who reads this book is going to die someday. If you want to live forever, maybe you should be praying—not depending on doctors, hospitals, technology and drugs.

3

DIAGNOSING THE
HYPERTROPHIC GREED GLAND

Health-care providers, particularly physicians, enjoy our greatest respect and admiration. We literally and willingly place our lives in their hands. In return, we expect them to conduct themselves nobly. They should be altruistic, professional, and beyond ethical and moral compromise. Fortunately, the vast majority of doctors and other health-care professionals strive for those standards, and it will always shock and frighten us to discover that there are those who don't.

While almost all humans possess a "greed gland" in some form, the term "hypertrophic" used in the chapter title refers to the abnormal enlargement of that tissue to the point that it's diseased and the stories describe pathological greed for money, admiration, status or other forms of satisfaction.

I graduated from medical school thinking I had joined the most humanitarian peer group in the world. Private practice has made me rethink my role as a physician. I quickly realized that the values and priorities were not universal in medicine. Medicine is a business populated by good and bad people. Surgeons slice you up with their knives and inflict pain. If somebody knifes you on the street, the cops are after him. I know, most would say it's entirely different. Don't bet on it. Sometimes what happens in the hospital is not any different than what happens on the street. In both cases, the man with the knife wants your money—and he might be willing to risk killing you for it. Let me warn you, if you think the hospital will police the doctor, you better hire a body-guard for yourself.

P hysicians are all bright and intelligent men and women. They all know the difference between good and bad medicine. Unfortunately, I've seen it too often, some will allow greed and ego to compromise their moral and ethical value systems. There's an overabundance of rules and regulations designed to control irresponsible professional behavior, but you can always find a loophole to nourish greed if you want it bad enough. These people can always justify their actions.

I don't think people want to believe it, they just don't want to believe that a doctor would do anything that wasn't in their patients' best interests. It's like questioning someone with higher authority. We are always taught to look up to people with higher authority, like doctors. And what people don't realize is that they are just as vulnerable and human as the rest of us are. They do all kinds of things they shouldn't do.

I 'm convinced that the future of medicine is under a dark storm cloud because of the actions of a few but significant number of practitioners. And many of the technical advances we've seen are prime sources for unjust enrichment by the greedy.

Everything in medicine has improved, except the unspoken standards of ethics. As medicine has expanded, so have the number of ethical issues. Unfortunately, medical schools and other health-related institutions have not been able to adequately address the issue of personal standards of ethics. Government has not been effective in changing the practice behavior of individual health-care providers. National, state and local medical societies lack legal authority to control behavior. Hospitals are hesitant to act because all physicians react negatively to policing. They're afraid innocent people may be indicted along with the guilty, and those kind of charges never disappear from the record.

Word of mouth builds medical practices. Word of mouth also sends patients to other doctors. Word of mouth destroys medical practices. The bad guys have aggressive attorneys who can easily scare off the good guys. If hospitals' management and medical staff officers get too aggressive in the area of ethics, most of the doctors will admit their patients to another hospital. So the bottom line is, unscrupulous physicians tend to be tolerated by their peers, hospitals and the government as long as they are not killing patients. Even then, if the press doesn't hear about it, not much is done.

It's this very tolerance of unethical behavior that's the prime cause of out-of-control costs. The only control we've seen has been increased bureaucratic regulations. That doesn't stop the bad guys, it only impacts on the good people.

I think we've all known a few physicians whose lives were controlled by a gland never found in an autopsy—the greed gland. This gland is found somewhere between the brain and the testes. Usually you'll find it in a GP or a family practice physician with a big referral network. This type of physician is like a pimp who solicits clients for prostitutes—the specialists. He abuses customers and shares them with whores under his control, who like himself are primarily interested only in a large, fast fee. There is no emotional bonding with the customer. There is no respect, only covert contempt. "Do the job fast, satisfy the client quickly and get away from the customer as soon as possible," that's the whore's motto.

I think most physicians are decent, honest and ethical people who devote their lives to treating the sick and the infirm. Unfortunately, every physician has the misfortune of being painted by the same brush used to expose the greedy members of the medical community. It is impossible for medical schools to consistently screen out applicants who might be less than desirable.

There is no simple ethics or moral screening test. You can check for a criminal record. You can ask for personal letters of reference. The truth is, unethical people are usually very bright and devious individuals whose innate cunning protects them from exposure. Maybe simple vocabulary tests would help because sometimes words have tricky spellings or pronunciations. How can one predict whether a medical student applicant can distinguish between the words "Hippocratic" and "hypocritic"?

The attitudes of doctors have changed dramatically. Many of them give up before they start. It goes back to the governing agencies—they're driven by them, too. They get upset when they have to send their patients home when they don't think it's time. They can't even order the medications they want because Medicare and Medicaid and HMOs won't pay for certain drugs. They get very upset.

And, it makes the good doctors, the ones who really care about their patients, devious. They have to find ways to get around all those frickin' limitations. They learn what to write down and when to write it down and how to say it. It doesn't matter what the government tries to do in reforming health care, the doctors are going to have to try to figure a way to get around it so they can treat the patients the way they know they should.

I 've got some statistics right here to give you an idea of the scope of the problem. In 1991, there were 6,634 hospitals in the United States with a total of 1.2 million beds that admit almost 34 million patients a year who stay an average of nine days per admission. That translates into over 300 million days of hospitalization. In 1991, there were over 400 million outpatient visits. By the year 2000 national health spending will increase to $1.6 trillion or sixteen percent of the GNP. Conservatively, it is estimated that ten percent of the services provided are medically unnecessary. That translates into $80 billion in the early 1990s and $106 billion in seven years. Effective controls for fraud and abuse will provide all the money that is needed to insure universal health care for all Americans.

Now, another frightening hypothesis suggested by health-care insiders is that twenty percent of all surgeries performed are unnecessary. Can you imagine the human pain and suffering resulting from greedy physicians and other providers?

Here's some more on that. In 1991, 23 million surgeries were performed in the United States. The cost of those surgeries is estimated to range from $115 billon to $230 billion. That's fourteen to twenty-eight percent of health care expenditures. If twenty percent of those surgeries were unnecessary, then $11.5 billion to $23 billion was wasted and went into someone's pocket. I think this demonstrates that there is an enormous feeding chain by health-care providers in unnecessary surgeries. Most of those who benefit do not even question the surgeries. They just take the money.

What is the feeding chain in unnecessary surgeries? Here's a simple, but not complete list. These are the people who earn money—the surgeon, the assistant surgeon, the anesthesiologist, the radiologist, the laboratory physician director, the medical directors of all other special hospital departments (such as respiratory therapy—where the doctor even gets a percentage of the oxygen used), all the other special doctor consultants such as cardiologists and neurologists (to name two), the hospital, the drug companies, the medical supply firms, the malpractice insurance agencies, and the contracted business services. One surgery provides income for every one of these.

And unnecessary surgeries are just the tip of the medical abuse system. Similar activities and opportunities exist in every aspect of health care. It's the way the game is played. Medical ethics, even in religious hospitals, leaves a great deal to be desired.

When I took this job as the administrator, I started to look at various activity reports. Two in particular—the census list and the surgery schedule. The census list because not only did it tell me how many patients were in-house, but what doctors were admitting them. The surgical list was important because that's where we make our money, the greatest revenue in the shortest period of time.

It didn't take long to recognize one surgeon's name operating every day, all day long. Every surgery was a circumcision, and what really made me curious was that every patient had a Vietnamese name.

Upon investigation, I found that the community had a very large population of Vietnamese refugees who, either by lack of custom or the civil war, still had their foreskins intact. These guys wanted to be "Americanized," so they went to a doctor who just happened to have an arrangement with this surgeon I mentioned. The surgeon would give the referring doctor $50 in cash for each referral, and then he'd bill $200 for the surgery. This was so successful he bought a bus to pick up the patients in the morning and return them home several hours later.

Profitable? You bet! He could do three surgeries an hour with ease, and he kept the patients coming all day long. That's $450 an hour, $3,600 a day, $18,000 a week, and with a month off for vacation a year, I figured he grossed $864,000. Not bad for a snip here and there with no major responsibility for medical follow-up, that was the referring doctor's responsibility. Of course, the referring doctor did quite well too—almost a quarter of a million dollars.

And who paid for all this? You and I did. Most of these patients had all qualified for state medical assistance, and circumcisions were approved without question.

One day a pathologist came into my office, obviously with something on his mind. He was extremely polite and started by saying, "We have a problem." It's always "we" when doctors talk about problems with the administrator.

It seems certain influential doctors on the hospital's medical staff decided that they needed to increase their income. They arranged to open a medical laboratory to compete with the hospital's lab for office and outpatient testing. To be licensed by the state, such a lab would need a qualified director, and they wanted someone who wouldn't question unnecessary testing and over-utilization.

They chose this pathologist. He was offered a minimum salary and a small percentage of the profits. At first he declined, but he was told to cooperate or else they would see to it that he lost his job at the hospital. In addition, his wife owned and managed a good restaurant in town, and it was implied the place would be boycotted. The doctors involved had the influence to make the threat real. They really had him by the balls, and being a pacifist and a foreigner put him at a real disadvantage.

Finally, after much circling around the problem, he said he had to unwillingly participate against his better judgment, but he was powerless to do otherwise. There was a lot of money to be made, and the public would never know they were being ripped off. He left my office thinking he had absolved himself of any blame.

I worked with a radiologist a few years back who insisted that only one manufacturer made acceptable film for x-rays. He claimed it was super-fast film which would reduce radiation exposure to the patient. He was extremely obstinate about having only this film in the radiology department.

Now I happen to know that drug and medical supply companies spend millions on convincing doctors that their products are the best. Some doctors agree with the claims and demand a certain product, like this guy I'm talking about. However, a few doctors use this opportunity to accept money from the manufacturing rep, who always appreciates getting the business.

As the department head, I knew of another manufacturer of super-fast film which happened to be much, much cheaper. This radiologist insisted that this particular brand was unacceptable. He claimed that the film he wanted was also clearer and reduced the number of repeat examinations. So we put it to a blind test and switched film without him knowing it. You guessed it. He liked the cheaper film better. Not long afterwards, another radiologist told me I had cut off the other's slush fund. Within a few months, I was looking for another job.

We had a cardiologist on staff who ordered every test that we had equipment in the department to perform on every patient he admitted or was a consult on. Some of these procedures were obsolete by technical standards, but he still ordered them.

I guess what bothered me and the other techs the most about it was that we'd have to scramble to get these done before the patient was discharged, and then it would take him two or three weeks before he'd come in to look at the results. I can see three possible benefits from this method of diagnosing. The first is to the patient; however, since the patient was usually discharged by the time the doctor saw the tests, that benefit remained only a possibility.

The other two were more direct and concrete. One, the doctor got a fee for interpreting the tests regardless of whether they helped the patient or not. And two, if he ever wound up in court, he had plenty of documentation that he did everything he could for the patient.

I worked in a doctor-owned hospital in which the medical director of the cardiopulmonary department was one of the major owners of the hospital. He made sure that every possible test was ordered that could possibly be ordered when a patient was admitted because not only did he get a cut as medical director of that department, he also got another cut when it came time to divvy up the hospital profits at the end of the year.

I still believe that ninety-five percent of the physicians that we do cardiac testing for are legitimate. I really believe that. But there is five percent out there who aren't. We had one doctor who had lots of patients in convalescent homes—this happened a couple of times—he'd order a test on a patient and our diagnostic service would go to the convalescent home and discover that the patient had died a few weeks before. We'd call the office and let his nurse know. Several weeks later he'd call and scream at us because we didn't do the test. Hey, we wanted the business as much as he did, but you can't do much on a dead patient.

O ne of my accounts is an orthopedic surgeon who has three locations in the county. Each one has a connecting side that does pain management, basically giving injections for pain, that they refer a patient to if after they've operated on them the pain continues. Well, this orthopedic surgeon also owns an MRI scanning service. Not every patient gets a Magnetic Resonance Imaging ordered when they come to him on the orthopedic side, unless they really need it. But if it can't be justified, he sends them to the other side of the building for pain management. Maybe there, they'll do an MRI. If not, and they determine there's nothing that they can do for them on that side of the building, then they refer them back to the orthopedic surgeon. He then refers them to the MRI scanning service. No matter what, he's got a pain management center and a referring physician on the other side that just keeps bouncing them back to him. Eventually they get an MRI. He's making money every step of the way.

W eight loss is big business for doctors. A big, big thing. I have a doctor who has a weight clinic, and he prescribes medication on a weekly basis for his patients. These gals, and men too, go in and pay fifty bucks a week to get a package of fourteen pills. He buys a thousand of them for $14 from me. A thousand. He turns around and charges $50 to the patient to come in and get a package of fourteen pills. You start doing the arithmetic on that, and he's making over $3,500 profit on those thousand pills that cost him $14. Then thrown in on top of that, he charges for the physicals, the prephysicals, the lab work and everything else.

W hen a doctor is in the market for a piece of equipment, I know for a fact that ninety percent of them are looking at three or four different manufacturers. And sometimes it's up to ten. I've been in situations where I've had to compete against ten different manufacturers to get the order.

Here's another scam they pull on us that's related to that. They'll want us to come in and do a demo for them. That's fine, we'll do the demo. We'll do two or three patients. What we find out later is, they're billing those tests. We as manufacturer's reps are doing demos on their patients, and they're billing out and getting reimbursed. They don't even own the equipment. They haven't even purchased it yet. Now, they'll bring in reps from four or five manufacturers. We all do the same thing, so for two or three weeks they're getting free testing and charging $300 a test. So what is that, fifteen free ultrasound tests at $300 a shot? That's $4,500 that they can collect without a penny of investment.

I sold a doctor four holter monitor recorders. I delivered them and instructed him and his staff in how to operate them, and then said, "Thanks. I'll see you later." He grabbed me by the elbow and said, "Oh, no, no. We're going to hook up some patients." I said, "You don't have any scheduled. That's what your staff said." He said, "Just a minute."

He walked out to the waiting room and said, "You. You. You. And you. Back in here." We hooked up all those patients. I guess if a doctor wants to hook somebody up, he just does it. He can always figure out a way to justify it to the insurance carriers. You think he didn't bill for them? He billed for all of them. That's what his nurse told me later. Now there's a bad apple.

I f you take a look at some of the private practice physicians that have x-ray equipment, chest x-ray units or things like that, what you find is that the quality of those pieces of equipment is low. They're either cheap equipment or very, very old and not maintained properly. The doctor listens to their chest and hears some congestion and says, "Hmm, you need a chest x-ray." Or a person comes in with a wrist that hurts. "Well, I better take a picture of this and take a look."

Then what happens is you can't make a diagnosis because the films are such poor quality, and the patient ends up having another study of proper diagnostic quality at the hospital or a clinic. Not only do these guys do this and it may be marginally ethical, but they're doing it and not even upholding the quality standards of a good hospital that's encumbered by the Joint Commission on Accreditation Health Organizations review and all of that. Private practice physicians don't have the same quality standards. And even if the films are nondiagnostic, that doesn't prevent the patient from being charged for them.

I think the tragic part is, they need to be policed. The only ones really policing the medical profession these days are the lawyers. And they're not doctors. They don't know medicine.

A surgeon was doing gall bladder surgery on a middle-aged guy, and during the operation, his nurse said, "Doctor, the blood pressure's dropping on your patient." The doctor stopped everything and looked at his anesthesiologist. "Is everything OK?" he asked, and the anesthesiologist said, "Yes," so he went back to work.

About four minutes later, he's about to close the guy up and the nurse hits him in the ribs and says, "Your patient's dead." Everything was flatline. He looks over at the anesthesiologist who's got earphones on. It turns out he was listening to a baseball game and wasn't paying attention to the patient. The patient's wife and children were told, "It's terribly unfortunate. He just had heart failure and he died." There was no formal medical staff follow-up. No nurses filed a complaint. Nothing was done to the physician.

Yesterday, when I was going to reveal that story at a Kiwanis meeting, I told it to a doctor beforehand. His first comment was, "That's done every day. Those guys get bored."

We were in the center of a malpractice trial. We had a neurosurgeon, an orthopedic surgeon and an anesthesiologist that were going to testify as to the disabilities of our client. However, we settled the case that morning, so by lunch time we were done. We were walking out of the courthouse, and since we were paying for them all day long, we said, "Come on, let's go to lunch." Well we were talking about the case, and it got around to three o'clock in the afternoon and those clowns were still drinking. We were all feeling pretty high, and we went from talking about the case to talking about standard of care. The doctors were kind of talking among themselves and then, I'll never forget this, one doctor turns to another, and he says, "How many have you killed?" Without even a hesitation, the other said, "Six." And then he turned right around to the third one, "How about you?" He said, "Four." Then the two who had been asked turned on the anesthesiologist and said, "How about you?" He said, "Only two that I know of."

I'm sitting there listening to this and I said, "What do you mean? Were you sued in all those cases?" One doctor said, "Are you crazy? Hell, no." I said, "How come you weren't?" He said, "It was just one of those things that happened."

Then the lawyer part of us got to talking about the equities of that and the conscience of it. To them, they deal with death every day. It wasn't a big deal. But these were cases where admittedly in their own consciences they had screwed up badly. There's no policing of that. Unless you're a doctor, you're not going to be privy to that type of locker room talk.

I'm an insurance investigator. The most fascinating case I ever had involved a young man. He had taken his girl on a date and was driving home in his Volkswagen bug when another car, a big Chevrolet full of high school kids, went through a stop sign and hit him broadside. As they hit him, the right front door swung open and he was thrown out the right side of the car, at least as far as his shoulders. When the car rolled, he injured his spinal cord. They took him to the hospital and determined he was quadriplegic. From the neck down—couldn't move. He was a senior in high school.

We got the case just that way. The insurance company for the kid who ran the stop sign offered $10,000. That was their policy limit in those days. Well that's a drop in the eye for a quad, so the parents went to an attorney. He said, "That's all the money there is from the kids that ran the stop sign, but let's hire an investigator and see if there's any other responsibility anywhere."

So I started the case and went to the scene. My first thought was, maybe the stop sign had been knocked down, wherefore you have city responsibility. Number two, maybe somebody worked on the brakes before the accident, and the brakes failed, that's what the driver of the other car had said. I checked a few other things like that, and had no luck. I went back to the attorney and told him I didn't see any other way. It was just an idiot kid running a stop sign. The parents took the $10,000.

I don't know why but the case stuck in my head, I guess because of the horrendous injury. The kid was getting straight As in school, and he was going to be an accountant; the family was a magnificent family.

Anyway, on my birthday, which was about nine months later, I don't know why it was, it's never happened before or since, in the middle of the night, I was wide awake thinking about that case and was wrestling it around in my head. Stop sign was up. Brakes were OK. Could there be anything else? Then my brain told me, "You stupid fool, you've looked at everything up to the time of impact but just stopped there."

The thought was, when did he become totally paralyzed? Was it at impact? Then I thought, wait a minute. There's some responsibility to the ambulance. Did they sandbag him? On a spinal cord injury, you've got to make the shoulders and spine immobile to prevent further injury to the spinal cord.

When I checked that out, I found they hadn't sandbagged him. He had been taken by ambulance to the hospital with the driver of the other car, who was also badly injured. The driver of the other car remembered that they hadn't sandbagged him.

They had taken him to the county hospital because that was closest. When they went through the kid's wallet, they found out that he was insured, and the neurosurgeon who was called in said, "Transfer him to the other hospital, because then I can get paid. Over here I'm paid just as a county employee."

By the way, the neurosurgeon had been at a party and showed up at the hospital drunk. We were able to prove that he had been drinking all evening. Suddenly the case started to open up. There was responsibility for this quad. It went to the ambulance company and it went to the doctor for being on duty intoxicated.

The boy had been transferred to another hospital, so we took a look at the emergency room chart of the county hospital. It was really hard to read so we blew it up to about three feet by four feet so we could read the signatures and notes. It showed that the emergency room nurse had signed out that the boy had gone with a different ambulance company from the county hospital to the private hospital. When I went to see her she wasn't working anymore, she had some time off to have a baby.

I went to her house, and I told her what I was there for. "I just want to check out what happened at the emergency room, and I know you're not going to remember, but the boy was transferred to another hospital." Her first comment was, "I've been waiting for you to call." This was two years after the accident. She invited me in and told me to sit down.

She told me they put in those ice pick things that go into your skull to immobilize your spine. Apparently, they fell out on the way down the hall to the ambulance. I said, "Is that all?" She said, "No,"—none of this is in the medical records of course— "the poor kid fell off the gurney because they didn't have him strapped down." Then she said, "If you don't believe me, see the attending intern at the emergency room. His initials are right next to mine."

Sure enough, there were his initials. She couldn't remember the doctor's name, so I went back to the hospital and said, "Do you happen to know what this name is?" They told me they didn't. I went down to medical records. On the way, I took my coat off and grabbed a chart so I looked like a doctor or something, and I asked, "Who is this right here?" The librarian said, "Oh, that's so-and-so. Don't you remember him?" I said, "Oh, yeah. Where is he now?" "He's over in Arizona somewhere." The medical association gave me his address. He lived in some little town south of Phoenix.

I got him on the phone. I said the same thing I did to the nurse. "Remember this case? I know you probably don't because it was so long ago." He said, "Oh, yeah. That's the one where they dropped him off the gurney." We owned an airplane and I said, "I'm going to be in your area tomorrow if that's OK." He said, "Oh, yeah, sure, come on in anytime."

Again, the whole test was, was he paralyzed at the impact, or was he paralyzed at the fall from the gurney? They could have dropped him all they wanted to if he was already paralyzed. See, the whole case had to hinge on that.

So the attorney and I flew over there and we met with him. He remembered most of it. "Well, I'll tell you this," he said, "when I first saw the kid in the emergency room, there was a screen around him because we didn't think he was going to live. He was having a hard time breathing so we called a Catholic priest in."

Here's another wild coincidence. The Catholic priest happened to have been my algebra teacher in high school. He had just retired and was the hospital chaplain. So I called him. I said, "Did you give this kid the last sacraments?" and he said, "Yeah." I said, "Could you see his feet moving?" He said, "Yeah, his feet were jerking." Then he said, "And the kid blessed himself."

Now you can't bless yourself and be paralyzed. You just can't. Your arms just don't work. Maybe after six or eight months with a little regeneration, you might be able to do something, but not then.

The doctor thought he remembered the feet jerking, but wasn't all that positive. We had the feet jerking and we had the Sign of the Cross. The doctor said, "There's a lot more to this, I'm sure." He was into hypnotism as a recall device so we flew him up to Carmel, California to the top guy in the nation on this. I was there when they hypnotized him. It was the darndest thing. We had to record it all so we weren't planting things in his head. We were letting him tell his story.

When we put him under, the first thing he started to do was laugh. We said, "How come you're laughing?" He said, "Well, while they're giving him Last Rites, his mother is standing over against the wall with her husband. She must have dressed awfully hurriedly because she's got on one of her husband's socks and she's got on these furry slippers that are like bear feet. She looks awful funny."

Then he confirmed the moving of the feet, and the reflexes were all there. He relived the entire thing, you could just see it in his expressions. As they were pushing the gurney down the hallway, just when they got to where they were going to lift the gurney up onto the ambulance, they lost the gurney and it tipped. You could just see him jump as he was reliving the memory of it. Then he put the kid back on. As he relived when the ambulance drove away, he just goes like this, he buries his head, figuring it's out of his jurisdiction.

After that, I played the tape to the mother of this boy. She remembered she'd put on her husband's socks, of all the stupid things.

So here you've got a case that suddenly is worth giant money because of the terrible negligence all around. Of course everybody denied everything. There was cover-up every step of the way. But we had done our homework and we privately went to the judge and told him what we had.

The sad part was, we went to trial. It took us all day to pick a jury. In those days you had to be allowed to raise your demand. The judge was so impressed with our facts that he raised the demand from $100,000 to a million. The next morning, we were ready to start the trial, and the boy died of a kidney infection. We ended up with about $120,000 in medical. That's all we could collect. If the patient dies, all you can recover is the medical expenses.

The kid was dead. The neurosurgeon went scot-free. He wasn't disciplined by anybody. And you know what? He was mad at us! He was so mad that we even questioned his integrity.

About one in five hundred abortions, even when they're performed in a hospital, one in five hundred goes wrong. That's a pretty high percentage, but I have yet to handle a malpractice trial for a fouled up abortion. Why? I think because the client is usually embarrassed to even admit to the outside world that she was pregnant, so those cases just die. And a good percentage of the doctors doing abortions are getting paid under the table. Many of the doctors aren't insured, so they sure aren't going to admit to any problems.

One of the worst physicians I've encountered was a vascular surgeon. I first became aware of him when a pulmonary medicine specialist came storming into my office, angry that this doctor had performed a certain surgical procedure that he defined as "mayhem." He charged that the doctor had willfully and permanently destroyed a patient's ability to survive. After the protesting physician calmed down, he explained that a questionable procedure was done on a patient with emphysema. It consisted of severing the carotid nerve on both sides of the neck. The function of this nerve is to alert the brain of a shortage of oxygen and the excess of carbon dioxide. Without this function, a person would never be warned of impending unconsciousness. If the patient were to drive to higher altitudes, he could possibly blackout because he wouldn't have a warning system for oxygen deprivation. Such a driver of a car on a mountain road would have a great chance of a fatal crash. Nobody would suspect the cause of death. The surgeon's greed would be buried with the patient.

Apparently, this doctor found his potential surgical victims by visiting rural areas searching for emphysema patients. He would give free public lectures, and his snake oil was a film showing the before and after effects of the surgery. The film would begin with a patient slowly walking, attached to an oxygen tank on wheels. The patient would next be seen getting off the surgery table and dancing down the hallways. A miracle had happened, and for only $15,000, it could happen to anyone who wanted it.

What the patient didn't know was that overexertion would probably kill him. This doctor was a con artist, but his patients saw him as a sort of faith healer or miracle worker. Patient testimonials were recorded on film within hours of surgery. The result was a dramatic sales and marketing program that appealed to desperately and terminally ill people.

Once he made the sale, he would bring these new patients to the big city from small farming communities throughout the Midwest. Of course, the surgery was performed with full payment in advance. The hospital stay was two days and the recovery would be uneventful. The simple surgical procedure would last only fifteen minutes, and the patient would only be mildly sedated. The patient would return home, never to be seen again. A consultation note was never sent to the patient's doctor back home, medical follow-up was never suggested. Money just flowed and flowed into his bank account. After returning home, patients could have sudden death from overexertion, and the cause would never be found on a routine autopsy.

He came to our hospital because it was small. Large hospitals are usually controlled by medical specialists who sharply criticize and prevent questionable procedures. I asked the pulmonary medical specialist to call for a special meeting of the medical staff executive committee to discuss the carotid nerve resection procedure, which he did. The meeting turned into a fiasco of surgeons and internists fighting over turf. The surgeons resented the internal medicine specialists getting involved in their area of expertise. The surgeons saw nothing wrong with the procedure. Their main concern was that the pulmonary medicine specialist was a professor at the local medical school and this was a town-and-gown versus private-practice physician dispute. Nothing was resolved except the doctor didn't admit any more patients to our hospital. He just moved on with his patients to another one. Since no disciplinary action was taken, it was not required to report the problem to the state medical board.

Several weeks passed without discussion of the issue, then the pulmonary doctor stepped into my office. He said, "The first patient that was operated on is dead. His car went through the guardrail on a high mountain pass. That patient and his entire family are dead. No one knows who was driving. Your insurance carrier is lucky!"

Nobody on the medical executive committee wanted to follow-up on the case. I was advised to forget it because this was a professional jurisdictional problem. Several years later while watching television, there on the screen was this same doctor watching one of his patients dancing down a hospital corridor to the applause of family and employees. The announcer praised the miracle that was being witnessed. The world was being told that emphysema patients could be freed from bondage to the oxygen tank.

The postscript to this story is that the doctor interested a research physician at a major medical school in experimenting with the surgical technique. That researcher was only interested in having live patients to treat like research animals and getting grants and publishing papers. Having found a willing partner to provide a shield of respectability for his greed, the doctor could tell his unsuspecting potential victims that he was a member of the research attending staff of one of the nation's most prestigious medical schools and teaching hospitals. In time, the pulmonary specialist who had warned of the doctor's activity was successful in scientifically discrediting the procedure. This doctor no longer cuts a patient's throat for money.

This is one of the biggest cases I ever worked. I'm not sure the guy is still alive, but he should be. He was drunk on the freeway and was in an accident. He had hit a parked car on the side of the freeway.

Anyway, he had a lower back injury. They yanked him out of the car and put him in an ambulance and took him to the county hospital. The accident was only a couple of blocks away. They didn't immobilize him; they didn't really examine him for three or four hours because he was drunk. Now he's paralyzed from the waist down. In that case we had problems with the drinking, of course, but again we had to determine when he had the spinal cord injury. Was he able to move his feet? When was the spinal cord injured? Did they sandbag him? In that case, we needed to know.

Immediately when he came into the hospital, he had had x-rays and those x-rays would have told us about the displacement and help verify when he was injured. We needed to find that out. First we sent a messenger and they said, "We can't find them." So after two or three of those attempts, which is often normal, I went in and said, "I have a subpoena here and I want the records. The medical records clerk looks though the files and comes back and says, "Sorry, I can't find them."

Well, there was a guy standing there who looked like her boss, and I went over to him and I said, "I need these really bad," and I told him why. "This kid's paralyzed and we're trying to determine, was he paralyzed at the scene and what's the condition of his spinal cord? The x-rays will show that." He said quietly, "Would you like to go for a cup of coffee?" I said, "Yeah." He said, "No, not today. I'll call you."

A day later he calls me and says, "Come on, I'll meet you at such-and-such." It was about ten miles from the hospital where he worked. When I met with him the next day, he said, "Let me tell you something. X-rays all have a code number, like '26-412.' What we do when we know a case is going to go to trial, where we know we were wrong, we'll deliberately file it a hundred above. That way, when someone asks for the correct number and we look in the proper place in the files, it's not there. We can say, 'take a look yourself, there's nothing there.' " I went back with my subpoena, and sure enough, there it was, right where he said it would be.

In a malpractice case—*mal* means bad—the only one that can say bad practice is another doctor. What we see today in the malpractice verdicts is just terrible. A lot of times they're very good cases that should have been filed and settled for a lot of money, but the doctors hang together where no one will testify against another in malpractice.

This case went down the drain because we couldn't get a doctor to testify against the doctor who committed malpractice.

A mother of nine kids—she lived in Pomona, California. She went to the doctor with a bad stomachache on a Monday. The doctor examined her and said, "No, you'll be all right." He gave her some pills and instructed her to come back Wednesday if she was still hurting. That's the standard of care.

She came back Wednesday and she was doubled over and she could hardly move. The doctor examined her and said, "We better get you into the hospital for some tests." It was about nine o'clock in the morning. He said, "Get a toothbrush, get in there this afternoon, and I'll come and see you." So he called over to the hospital and made the bed reservation, but because he had an office full of patients, he forgot about it.

So the gal checks into the hospital, but they don't know what's wrong with her. The doctor didn't show up that afternoon. He went on a vacation. He went fishing. Friday, the mother died of a ruptured appendix, leaving nine kids orphaned.

It was two-fold in stupidity. The doctor screwed up. He should have treated his patient. Going on vacation and forgetting about your patient is below the standard of care. The real tragedy though was the complete stupidity of the nurses. They said, "What could we do? We couldn't treat this patient. We didn't know what was wrong." Well, I could tell you what to do, get yourselves a doctor and find out! The gal was in excruciating pain and she died. There was no excuse for it.

When we went on that case representing nine little kids, we couldn't find a doctor that would say that was below the standard of care. We went all the way to San Diego looking for one.

Why? Because doctors feel like they're betraying one of their brethren, so they refuse. I'm sure there's a few hard-nosed guys that will call a shot the way it should be. But it's sad that there aren't more like that. You can't allow this kind of thing to happen.

They lost the case. We couldn't find an expert that would testify on standard of care. So without a doctor we couldn't win. The hospital settled. In law, they call it "momentary forgetfulness." Three days of it? That wasn't below the standard of care?

The doctor went scot-free. Scot-free. Nobody did a thing. Those kids are still wandering around, without a mother, without a father. Somebody should be responsible.

A stewardess was on an overnight. She was taking a shower the next morning before she caught her plane to go back home, and she noticed a lump in her breast. It was a pretty good sized one, and it scared her. The airline had a team physician, so she went and met the doctor at the hospital. He felt for the lump and it was there all right, so he said, "We're right here. Why don't we do a biopsy and we'll find out whether it's malignant or not?"

She hung around and they did the biopsy, and then the doctor came back in and said, "Well, I've got good news and bad news. The bad news is it's malignant. The good news is it's localized. If we do a mastectomy now, it'll be all right. The history on these is pretty good, so you'll be out of danger." So what do you do? She's twenty-two years old and she said OK. The next day, off comes the breast.

Well, when the doctor came into the recovery room, he was

extremely happy. He said, "Do I have good news for you. It wasn't malignant after all." I suppose a percentage of the people who got that kind of good news might say, "That's great." But she wasn't one of them.

The doctor blamed the hospital lab. Pathology said no way. We subpoenaed a copy of the pathology report ordered on that specific biopsy. They said, "Well, here it is. We gave it to the doctor saying there was nothing, and we gave it to him in time." Then it became a question of did he operate too soon. They pointed at each other. That will usually make the case deeper and more expensive to everybody. But you've got to remember that by fooling around like that, fifty percent of the really good cases are thrown away and lost.

This lady received a settlement but there was no disciplinary action taken against the doctor or the hospital.

F ive doctors got together. They were old buddies from medical school, and they would meet once a week and have lunch and compare Mercedes and golf clubs. They were all well to do. They were way up in their dollar-making and in their reputation, but they got bored.

During conversation, they might ask, "Did you do an operation this morning?" "Yeah, I did an appendectomy. What did you do?" "A tonsillectomy." One day just for fun, and apparently it was all innocent at the beginning of it, they said, "Well, tell you what. Let's each put a hundred dollars on the table, and then a week from now when we meet again for lunch, the one who's done the most appendectomies gets the pot." One week it was appendectomies, one week it was tonsillectomies, and one week it was gall bladders.

Along comes a week, and a patient saw one of the doctors for a severe stomachache. He had a history of ulcers. The doctor took out his appendix. When the patient asked, "Why did you do that? I've had an ulcer problem for the last ten years," the doctor said, "Well, this will improve that condition substantially. You watch."

Well it didn't do a damn thing. So the patient sued him, and as he sued him, this luncheon wager jumped out. I was investigating the case and I happened to know one of the nurses. She said, "Don't you know what you're into in this one?" I said, "Hell, no. What do you mean? This idiot just took out an appendix when he shouldn't have." She said, "Oh, no," and then out came the story. You should have seen those doctors run for cover. It never came out what was going on. The case was paid.

The insurance company didn't know about the other doctors and the weekly bet, the one doctor just sent a letter to his insurance company saying, pay this claim. He didn't have to say why, he just said pay it, and they did. An insurance company will pay a claim off of a doctor's letter. He'll talk over their heads saying, "Well, it was my professional opinion that because of the . . . blah blah blah." And once the money's paid, it's over. The only obligation that an attorney has to his client is that the client is fairly compensated.

The total disciplinary actions by state medical boards in 1991 was 3,034. Out of a total of 584,921 private practice physicians, only five percent were subject to disciplinary action. Most of the charges were for being impaired by drugs and alcohol, not malpractice, or unscrupulous or immoral behavior. That's ridiculous! I bet even a convent has a greater percentage of people needing discipline than that.

The president of the AMA on several occasions has pointed out that only about five percent of medical malpractice ever comes to light and only about ten percent of that is ever litigated. Of those that actually go to trial about forty-five percent will be successful, about fifty-five percent will not be.

Anybody who has any experience in the health-care field has seen malpractice, and most of the time the patient or the family was unaware of it, never did learn about it. It's not something that's brought to the center of attention. Sometimes there are very clear efforts to cover it up.

There were a number of studies based on going back and looking at hospital records that indicated that. This is from medicine itself saying we have a problem. There's a small number of

physicians that repeatedly make mistakes and commit malpractice. Every physician makes mistakes. They're human, they make
mistakes. Unfortunately, physicians look upon malpractice as
some sort of punitive system, rather than as a system to compen-
sate someone who has suffered an injury that should not have
happened. It's basically become more of an insurance type of system, but the physicians look upon it as punitive.

F ewer than one-half of one percent of our nation's doctors face
   any state sanctions each year. And yet, based on studies by
Harvard University and several others, plus a Department of
Health Education & Welfare Malpractice Commission report of
injury malpractice cases, an estimated 150,000 to 300,000 patients each year are injured as a result of doctors' negligence.
When you consider that there are only 3,000 disciplinary actions
a year, does it sound like the quality of care that doctors deliver is
being monitored appropriately by the medical industry?

M alpractice insurance carriers really are the only policing
   mechanism for doctors; be that as it may. I think it was a
1989 Tufts University study that found that physician-owned
malpractice insurers sanctioned about thirteen out of every 1,000
doctors they covered. They terminated policies of six out of every
1,000 policyholders in 1985 because of negligence-prone behavior, and they restricted the practice, or imposed other sanctions,
on another seven of every 1,000 doctors where care was found to
be substandard.

   If this combined rate of malpractice insurance terminations
and other sanctions by physician-owned insurance companies
were applied to all physicians in the US, the rate would be nearly
four times higher than the actual 1991 average rate of serious
disciplinary actions by state medical boards.

L awyers have magazines published that show right now
   they're disciplining thirty to forty lawyers a month. Of those,
probably ten have their licenses revoked for life. Lawyers will

fight each other and be very critical. When a guy steps out of line, they'll jump on him, sometimes even unfairly, but they'll go after him and take his license away. Even though it's lawyers policing lawyers, they have a pretty good system.

In the medical profession, when was the last time you ever heard of a doctor's license being pulled? Sure you might read it in the newspaper occasionally, but you don't read it in their magazines. They keep it all closed in. When they discipline a doctor, they'll "talk" to them.

Even when you see accusations of sexual misconduct, say psychiatrists who molest their patients, do they pull their license? Sometimes, I guess. But usually, the doctor will just transfer from one state, or jurisdiction, to another. How often do they yank their license for life?

I n the vast majority of malpractice cases, the moment the check is cut, it's over. It's extremely rare that any disciplinary action is ever taken against the doctor. At the most, the insurance company might cancel the doctor, but normally they won't do that either, they'll just raise the premium. If a doctor does get canceled, it's easy to go out and get it through another carrier, but the premium goes up considerably.

I suppose in some cases I'm an accessory to the crime. If a private-practice doctor is practicing shoddy medicine, and it has to be pretty bad for me to know, there's nothing I can do because I can't afford to turn people in. I'd be cutting my own throat. If I turn in my best account that provides thirty percent of my business, suddenly I'm out of business. And if that doesn't end it for me, when the doctors talk among themselves, there goes the rest of it.

I f anyone tries to tell you that the American Medical Association, or any other medical association, is policing their own, you've got a wolf in the hen house. Doctors seldom have a lot of friends other than other doctors. They hold together and they protect each other. You don't get into that clique unless you're a doctor and you've got your degree and your specialty and all that goes with it.

Remember the case about the infertility specialist in Virginia who tricked his patients? He misled a staggering number of patients through false pregnancies and miscarriages. He used hormone injections to trick some patients into believing that they were pregnant when they were not, and he used his own sperm in artificial insemination while lying about the source. One patient said she experienced seven supposed pregnancies and miscarriages under his care in a three-year period. Another patient was forty-six and suffering from blocked fallopian tubes was given hormone injections. She was told she was pregnant; he assured her that the child was developing normally. Months later she was told that her baby was dead and had been reabsorbed into her body. The number of children this physician fathered, if you could use that term, is unknown, but from the examination of his medical records the number must be staggering.

He was charged with fifty-two counts of fraud and perjury, but what did his peers deem as sufficient penalties for all of this physician's deceit and fraud? He agreed to stop practicing medicine and now conducts privately funded medical research in Utah.

I don't know if you can regulate unethical behavior. There are so many avenues for fraud . . . I wonder. The only way I can see it happening is if it comes from the inside. Doctors have to take the first step. If a doctor diagnoses cancer in someone, do they ignore it? I hope not. So when they see one of their fellow doctors behaving unprofessionally, wouldn't it be better to remove the cancer, rather than ignore it and allow it to grow?

Can a medical staff discipline itself? These superficial altruistic "bastards" are afraid of their own shadows and are nothing but cowards when it comes to challenging the behavior of their peers. I knew one doctor who was an alcoholic. It was around Christmas time, and I got a call one day from the nursing director telling me that a doctor was making rounds and he appeared to be drunk. So I ran to the last area he had been seen. Sure enough, I, too, thought he'd been sampling the Christmas spirits too much and too early in the day. He tried to tell me he was a diabetic and had missed breakfast. That might have worked, except then he told me the alcohol I smelled was a beer he'd drunk the night before and that everyone knows it takes a long time for that odor to leave. My response was instantaneous. I said, "Doctor, your medical staff privileges are immediately suspended under the Protective Action Clause of the Medical Staff Bylaws. Go to the doctors' lounge, and I'll arrange for someone to drive you home."

The next day, I called a special meeting of the medical staff executive committee and informed them of the problem. They agreed to have a hearing and the necessary paperwork was prepared. At the hearing a few days later, the physician pleaded the old "I'm a diabetic" case again. It didn't work any better with them than it did with me. He offered to resign from the staff. As I've seen in other cases, that would have been enough. That was the doctors' way of resolving the problem—just remove him from sight. But another physician said, "No, we don't want you to resign. We want to help you with your problem." The medical staff decided his practice associate should cosign all of his orders for the next ninety days. Even though I objected, I was ordered not to make a report to the state licensing board.

This was a well-reported case. An attractive 59-year-old woman accused her physician of sexually assaulting her during a routine medical exam. While the patient was alone in the examination room, the doctor came in and tried to sexually stimulate her with an ultrasound transducer and his fingers. The patient was frozen and unable to speak. After she dressed, she overheard the doctor telling his office clerk, "No charge for this one."

The patient stopped at the local hospital after the incident.

She was told that the examination was inappropriate and to report it to the local medical society. A month later she wrote and received a letter from the local medical society saying it found that the doctor had done a proper examination and that the doctor would be advised that he should have a female nurse witness all exams.

After the publicity, ten more women came forward to file complaints against the doctor. Why did the first lady wait so long to press charges? In her own words she said something like, "I feel so stupid talking about this. I'm fifty-nine and I was raised that you don't question doctors. They deserve respect. They know what they are doing and they won't harm you."

The patient filed a civil case and accepted an out-of-court settlement of $17,500. Was justice served? I don't think so. Women, men too, need to question doctors and stand up for themselves. Too many people try to pretend that these things don't happen.

We had a kindly old anesthesiologist at our hospital whose skills were rapidly deteriorating. In the operating room, patients were given so much anesthetic they literally were turning black. Our surgeons and all of us nurses were getting worried but were afraid to take corrective action other than using a different anesthesiologist. This wasn't a solution because it was a small hospital with much activity, and the problem doctor was usually the only one available.

We went to the hospital administrator with the problem. That was a hard thing to do because he, the anesthesiologist, was our friend. He had been good to us over the years. On top of that, this doctor's wife had mismanaged their financial affairs, and they didn't have much for retirement. But still, he was too dangerous to the patients, so we asked that he be asked to retire.

The administrator asked the medical staff executive committee to act, but nothing was done—out of loyalty, I guess. By this time, we saw a big drop in the number of surgeries scheduled. Surgeons were going to another hospital.

So how was it solved? Remember, he was very popular with the other doctors. The administrator used the malpractice crisis, and convinced him that insurance premiums were only increasing and it was time to retire. He offered him a staff job with a fair, but minimum, salary, and the anesthesiologist opened a weight control clinic.

I read where a former high-level official with the Department of Health and Human Services said, "If a surgeon was standing over my mother with a scalpel, and I had a choice between a crook that was competent and a very honest physician that was impaired by drugs, alcohol or age, I would choose the crook."

I'm going to sound very cynical saying this, but it's what I believe, based on my experience dealing with doctors. I think that eighty to ninety percent of them are using the system for their own gain. I'm talking about using their staff, using the system, using the hospitals, using the suppliers, and using the patients. I really believe that. Most of them are in it for the money.

They've been in a position to take advantage of the system and not be second-guessed. While for the rest of us, if we're not very good at what we do, we're out. Not true with doctors. If we're a crook in this business, if we try to take advantage of the system, there's enough controls on us, we're spotted quickly and we're gone. Not with doctors. We've always got somebody looking over our shoulder, and often it's a doctor.

4

THE PRIVILEGE OF MEDICAL
PRIVILEGES

To be entrusted with the life of another human being is an awesome responsibility, and it should be viewed as a privilege. However, thankfully rarely, at times that trust is seen as creating the opportunity for unjust enrichment. How can the patient know when this has occurred? Shouldn't there be swift and stringent means to police and discipline those who violate that trust?

There are "literally thousands" of medical privileges and probably the most important area of medicine needing reform, and probably the most difficult area to fix, is the one which revolves around the granting and monitoring of those privileges. While some reforms are occurring, these are being instituted slowly, in a piecemeal fashion. As of now, there are no adequate methods of discipline that function throughout the system, a problem felt keenly by many of those working in health care.

When we talk about medical privileges, there are literally thousands of them. Aspiration, biopsy, endoscopy, catheterizations, arterial puncture, venous cutdown, spinal taps, electrocardiogram interpretation, hemodialysis. Emergency care ranging from gunshot wounds, near-drownings, heart attacks, shock, burns, lacerations, aneurysms, fractures, allergies and on and on. Category IV privileges include allergy, cardiology, dermatology, endocrinology, hematology, gastroenterology, infectious diseases, psychiatry, pulmonary diseases, nephrology, oncology and rheumatology.

Obstetrics and Gynecology has over thirty distinct procedures. Orthopedic surgery privileges cover at least thirty specific procedures. Podiatry has over twenty. Pediatrics has nearly forty procedures. Every specialty and subspecialty has over thirty specific or general procedures unique to their field. Monitoring and proctoring each specialist is virtually impossible.

We're talking about specialization and the various boards of specialization. Even among those boards, whether you're a neurologist or a neurosurgeon means different things. A neurologist can be a psychiatrist, a neurologist, and he can be a neurosurgeon. There's probably several other minor areas as well. But just to be a neurologist doesn't make you a surgeon and doesn't make you a psychiatrist, and you can really screw people up royally either way if you don't do it right.

Who determines what type of surgery a doctor can perform? It's not the medical school. It's not the internship hospital. Not a state licensing agency. Not the American Medical Association. Not the state medical society. Certainly, not the hospital management. It's the individual hospital's medical staff, and they act like independent corporations. They determine how medicine is practiced in each hospital.

They can organize as a large committee of the whole, or as departments such as Surgery, Medicine, Pediatrics or Obstetrics. Or they can be organized as committees without regard to medical specialty. Small hospitals usually organize this way. And that's where the problem lies. General practice physicians can sit on the surgical committee and can approve surgical privileges for any doctor on staff. Maybe the decision is based on an examination of training and experience. Or, maybe it's just based on the needs of the hospital. If that's the case, doctors are permitted to perform complicated procedures without the benefit of adequate training.

Worse yet, when a doctor screws up, who do you think has review jurisdiction? That's right, the same guys who approved his privileges. Do you think they want it public that they screwed up in approving privileges? Of course not. So generally, nothing is done to restrict the offending doctor.

What can be done to correct the problem? The answer's simple to explain, but will be difficult to implement. Difficult because it violates the total autonomy that medical staffs enjoy. A national physician licensing board should be established. This would ensure that every doctor practicing in the United States would have to meet the same basic requirements. Secondly, when a physician is licensed, it should stipulate what medical and surgical procedures he is allowed to perform. This would be based on information provided by approved residency programs and would eliminate "special certificates" from one week vacation seminars. A physician's privileges would be determined by his ability, not by the needs of the hospital.

Rural communities, whether they be in the mountains, deserts or farm counties, frequently contribute to their problem of inferior medical care. A small town in search of a doctor often settles for a candidate who is poorly trained, in trouble elsewhere or both. A rural hospital's board of directors who has spent years and many dollars recruiting a physician can put tremendous pressure on a medical board to grant a license. Pressure from constituents can influence elected officials to add more pressure or look the other way. When the "savior" doctor delivers poor care, local officials look the other way.

First things first. Who decides what a physician can do in a hospital as far as types of surgical procedures? Who decides what medical procedures a doctor will be permitted to do? Can anyone treat diabetes, heart problems or kidney failure? Of course not. It is impossible for one physician to be expert in all diseases.

An organized medical staff is formed under the wings of the hospital articles of incorporation and bylaws. This medical staff is delegated authority to practice medicine within a hospital. Most states have laws preventing the corporate practice of medicine, so administrators and directors can only accept or reject recommendations made by the organized medical staff through the elected chief of staff. If that were not the case, laymen would be practicing medicine without the required education, experience and license.

The process for medical staff membership is simple. An application form is submitted detailing educational and professional experience. At least three professional references must be given. The hospital will then verify the physician's license, malpractice insurance, education and personal references. The national data bank will be consulted regarding additional background information. With the application, the physician will pay a nominal sum ($25 to $50) that is designated for the medical library or maybe a hospital social activity.

When the paperwork is completed, it will go to a medical staff credentials committee for review. If the application is found to be in order, it is then forwarded to other committees for delineation of privileges. This is where the potential problems begin.

Medical staffs are organized by departments or as a committee of the whole. When the staff is departmentalized, only surgeons can review and grant surgical privileges and only internists can review and grant medical, that's nonsurgical, procedures. Specialists tend to be much more conservative and dedicated in granting privileges to competitors. This has two opposing results—higher standards and fewer specialists on staff. When privileges are granted by the committee of the whole, there is less stringent review of qualifications. Frequently, decisions are made on the basis of the reviewing doctors getting more referrals.

Clinical privileges fall into four broad categories. Category I are uncomplicated medical or surgical illnesses or procedures presenting no serious threat to life. Category II are diagnostic or therapeutic problems with no immediate threat to life. Category III are complex or severe illnesses with a serious or potential threat to life, and Category IV are unusual complex diagnostic or therapeutic problems and/or immediately life threatening. Physician qualifications vary with each category, and there is an opportunity that higher categories of practice are given than are justified by training and experience.

Let me get into each category a little deeper. Category I privileges are for those conditions appropriate for any medical, osteopathic, dental or podiatric school graduate with little or no formal training other than an internship and/or one or two years of practice. Consultation must be obtained when doubt exists as to the diagnosis or when response to treatment is not readily apparent. This is the level that should be assigned to general practitioners who are not board-certified. This level can take care of minor problems but are not competent to handle severe illnesses. Physicians in this category are the "gate-keepers" of medicine. What they lack in medical skills they more than make up in bedside manner. Their rapport with the patients and family members tend to be excellent. They play the "Dr. Marcus Welby" role to perfection. From my experience I believe that doctors in this category tend to believe that they own you. They are your doctor and god forbid any other physician takes you away from his list of customers. That means war! Since they decide to whom the patient should be referred, doctors in this class have specialists kissing their butts in every way possible. In medical staff problems, specialists tend to avoid the discipline of or criticism of referring primary care physicians. These doctors can get any administrator fired with very little effort. After all, they are the main source of patient referrals to a hospital.

Category II doctors generally includes those conditions of Category I plus conditions and procedures of increased scope and complexity gained with postgraduate formal residency experience, or skills that have been gained and maintained through experience. These physicians are also expected to seek consultation when indicated. Generally, doctors in Category II are not eligible to take national specialty board examinations.

It's my opinion that Category I and II physicians pose the greatest danger for incompetence and greed. Doctors in these groups tend to have their privileges increased by attending educational seminars in exotic vacation spots. They'll go on skiing or resort holidays that includes a brief lecture and film presentation for which a certificate is awarded. The doctor returns to the hospital and requests additional privileges based upon the educational vacation. Lower quality hospitals routinely grant such requests. Then their practice on live patients begins until their skills are developed. The danger is that the doctor might develop the mechanical skills without any understanding of the pathology. He might be able to manipulate a flexible scope within the body, but cannot understand what he finds. Meanwhile the money keeps rolling in, right out of the patient's pocket.

If someone thinks that they or a loved one has a Category III or IV condition, they should get away from the Category I and II doctor as fast as they can. That is right to do so. One thing is certain—they're either going to harm the patient, or their pocketbook, or both. And the patient will often thank them for it.

Doctors in Category III treat conditions in Categories I and II and may act as consultants when indicated. Physicians in this category are formally trained and are eligible to take, or have passed, a national specialty examination. These physicians are competent with only occasional acts of negligence. Being part of the human race, they experience the same problems of drug and alcohol that are common to other educated groups. This group tends to have the greatest numbers of business entrepreneurs. That's to be expected. They tend to be better educated, be more ambitious, and often have more opportunities for unjust enrichment.

Category IV physicians should have the highest level of competence or technical skills within a given field and are qualified to act as consultants. Physicians with these privileges are expected to have formal training and experience beyond residency requirements and are considered to attain eligibility for board subspecialties. These are the highest trained and most qualified of all physicians. They usually practice only in teaching or all-services hospitals. Seldom would they be found in a hospital smaller than five hundred beds, and never in a rural hospital. These are the "super doctors." Usually they lack the bedside charm of the doctors in the other categories. Rarely are they subject to the medical disease of looking for the quick buck. They are more interested in their subspecialty than their bank account. They are so good, they don't have to play the game of referrals and consultations.

Patients seek them out and not vice versa. Unfortunately, the average person can't get an appointment to see them.

Do doctors fall exclusively into one category? Absolutely not! It is possible that a physician eligible for Category IV privileges in a subspecialty may be eligible only for Categories I, II or III in other fields.

OK, back to applying to the medical staff for privileges. Initial privileges granted by medical staffs are based upon interviews, recommendations of previous associates or instructors, monitoring of records, observation of techniques and other sources. Medical staff applicants should submit verifiable documentation of skills relating to patient selection, correctness of technique and patient outcome. Privileges are delineated, or specified, in each category and are assigned provisional or probationary status. New physicians are subject to peer review by current medical staff members.

Once privileges are delineated, every doctor is expected to be able to recognize his or her own limitations and request consultations where indicated. Consultations should be just that—an opinion being asked for and given, with suggestions for care made by the consulting physician.

L et's look at how the doctor's privileges are policed and disciplined.

After the privilege categories are determined, enforcement raises problems. It's easy to monitor surgical privileges. A surgeon cannot schedule a procedure for which he is not approved. One trick that Category I and II doctors use to get around restrictions on their privileges is to book a surgery for an approved procedure, and once the patient is opened up, do something else. In smaller hospitals this is frequently done; larger hospitals vigorously monitor results of surgeries. Surgeons watch competing specialists. Anesthesiologists are always comparing surgeons and keeping notes for future actions or protection.

Unfortunately, the patient stands a twenty percent chance of having an operation that could have been avoided. That is true in any size hospital, but the smaller the hospital, the less is the supervision. Thus the percentage of unnecessary surgeries can dramatically increase. Look at all of the uteruses that have been cut out without justification. How many tonsils have been snipped without cause? Lots!

Monitoring and controlling clinical privileges is far more difficult. In treatments on the general nursing floor the doctor can easily avoid restrictions. Only if there is a bad result is the case and the doctor subject to review. And doctors do not like to criticize their peers face-to-face in a committee meeting.

Occasionally a physician will file a complaint. Here is an example in a letter written by an emergency room physician to an attending doctor. This letter led to a review by the medical staff. It reads:

Dear Dr. — —,

You will recall that we had two telephone conversations on July 20th regarding a patient of yours. This elderly gentleman presented to the Emergency Room in desperate straits. He was badly dehydrated, lethargic and unable to ambulate. History revealed that he had been ill for two or three days with a headache, anorexia and vomiting to the point that he was unable to take his medications and had only consumed one glass of water in the 24 hours before I saw him. My evaluation determined that he had a pneumonitis in addition to his above problems. . . .

The logical endeavor was to admit him to the hospital. Here is where the difficulties started, because before you would authorize admission you wanted more tests despite my protestations that the tests would be irrelevant to the disposition. You insisted. The test results were predictably abnormal. And, so, more time and expense was expended. Then you refused to admit him. You wanted the ER to hydrate him and send him home. . . . You insisted that I transfer him to another city for a "pulmonary consultation."

You, then, obviously tried to intimidate me by asking how long had I worked in your community's ER. When informed that it was my first day, you responded with a "no wonder" which meant that I did not know your modus operandi and that I had better get with the program. You gave me the name of another doctor, and after a two-hour hiatus and several phone calls, I talked to the doctor who was covering for the doctor you wanted me to contact. There were three or four telephone conversations with him. He questioned the indications for transfer, wondering why the patient could not be admitted to our hospital. Eventually, he informed me that another hospital would accept him, but the patient may be returned if there were no compelling reasons for the transfer. Finally, I talked to the ER doctor at that hospital, who accepted the patient for evaluation. Copies of the workup were sent with the patient. All of this took part of the morning and all of the afternoon.

The management of this patient could have been very simple—just admit him and treat him appropriately and then you obtain whatever consults you wanted or needed. Here is a 90-year-old man with long standing COPD [chronic pulmonary lung disease—emphysema] who was toxic. Why did he need a "pulmonologist"? Are you an internist? Have you never encountered such a "complicated case" in all your experience? Is he not your patient? Do you not, maybe, have some responsibility and accountability for his current state of affairs? Aside from those questions, there is the issue that time was wasted in his needed therapy and the added expense of all the tests, repeat tests and transportation are simply not justified. How about the time that his relatives were reduced to waiting around—not knowing? How about the statement from you to his granddaughter, when she confronted you about his disposition, that you wanted a "neurological evaluation"? Now, maybe in my most benevolent mood, I would concede that this man could use a "neurological consult" at age 40, 50, 60, even 70 and beyond, but a man 90 years old with a toxic state from the complications of COPD is simply ridiculous. Where is the neurological problem? What happened to his pulmonic problem?

I have never come across someone like you in all my years of family practice and emergency room experience. Granted, I have encountered some real difficult personalities during the years, in my attempts to obtain the needed evaluation and care of the multitude of patients who have presented to me either in my office or the ER. You are special. Not only do you ignore your responsibilities as their doctor, but you are ignoring their family, you are ignoring the added expense, you are ignoring your own community hospital and, worse yet, you are ignoring the standards of our profession. Need I say more?

Yes! I do! There are other issues involved here. The ER staff dislikes and distrusts you. You have succeeded in intimidating them. They, and the ER director, do your bidding to the detriment of everyone. Who else have you alienated with your arrogant and callous attitude? How about your colleagues? How about the administrator and staff of the hospital? I know about the staff because word has it that you do this kind of behavior all the time. How about the doctors who don't do any surgery anymore in "your" hospital? How about the Hippocratic Oath?

Sincerely,

and then it's signed by the doctor.

In this case, the patient that this doctor was referring to died two weeks later at another hospital. The private doctor did not want to admit the patient for treatment. He thought that an intravenous solution could be given in the emergency room and the patient sent home. This went to the medical staff for review, and when the patient's case was reviewed, the executive committee refused to take action. They washed their hands of the dispute. Nothing happened. That's typical of many medical staffs, especially in smaller hospitals.

When a physician graduates from medical school and completes a one-year internship, he is eligible to take an examination to become a physician and surgeon. Those tests are administered by an agency of state government, not the AMA. When a physician does additional study in one of the specialties of medicine, he earns a postgraduate diploma. The procedures that are actually performed in a hospital are determined by the hospital's medical staff independently of the AMA, the medical schools and the state licensing boards.

Delineation of medical and surgical procedures, which means

permission to perform specific treatments, is done solely by a hospital medical staff. Most hospitals carefully verify the applicant's educational and experience credentials and do not award privileges that are not earned. Some hospital staffs are lax in their surveillance of physician members and will grant any request for privileges without a thorough background check. I know of some who have even ignored information if there was an opportunity to earn more money by hospital admissions and consultations.

There was an interesting case in which the medical board and the attorney general were slow to act. It involved a doctor who graduated from a reputable medical school in the Mid-west and interned in one of the finest teaching hospitals in the country. She moved to our area where she opened a practice but soon strange things started to happen. Her spouse left town. That wasn't so strange, because couples break up all the time. But then the doctor's behavior became erratic and suspicious. Our hospital refused to grant her medical staff privileges. The doctor initiated a lawsuit against the hospital in an attempt to compel them to grant her admitting privileges. Something in the doctor's background was sufficient not to want an association with her.

While waiting for the appeal meeting to begin, our hospital attorney was reading the newspaper of the larger neighboring city. Being an attorney, his eyes naturally searched for the police and court log. And there it was. The doctor had been convicted of driving under the influence and had been sentenced to fifteen days in jail. The doctor's attorney withdrew the appeal.

Suddenly more stories started to surface. The local pharmacists were getting concerned about her prescriptions. There were numerous reports about the doctor being drunk and disorderly in public. The ambulance attendants reported seeing the doctor running down the street nude. Then the doctor was brought into the local hospital's emergency room with a drug overdose. The illegal drug was confirmed by testing.

Patients reported that the doctor was acting strange in the office—stumbling, falling down and being incoherent. But yet, she still attracted patients because the costs were low, credit was accepted and house calls were frequent.

One day a patient came to the hospital demanding the results of her lab work immediately. She had an appointment with a plastic surgeon one hundred miles away, and the doctor we've been talking about had refused to give her the results of the physical exam and lab work. After a violent argument, the doctor gave in and hand wrote the requested information. The patient wanted to confirm the results of the lab work, so she came to the hospital.

We had no record of her specimen ever being sent to us. One of our laboratory technologists, on a hunch, searched the computer files for any other patient results for the same doctor. Miracle of miracles—an exact match was found. That was a statistical impossibility. What the doctor had done was use another patient's results. Our hospital notified the medical board of the possible unprofessional action.

Then the truth came out. For six years the doctor had been committing acts of incompetency. The medical board was aware of the situation. Many complaints from other health-care providers had been filed for over a period of six years. No disciplinary action had ever been taken.

The failure to protect the public is universal. Some states are worse than others, but one thing is certain, the system doesn't protect the consumer from the incompetent or the impaired physician. Too little discipline is being done. Only one-half of one percent of the nation's physicians face any sanctions each year. Approximately 3,000 disciplinary actions are initiated every year. This is a pittance compared with the hundreds of thousands of patients who are injured or killed each year in hospitals alone as the result of medical negligence.

Doctors make the mistakes and the good doctors don't want to be involved in reporting or testifying because of the retaliation by legal terrorists. The number of serious disciplinary actions indicates either a cover-up or incompetency on the part of hospital medical staffs, ignorant hospital boards of directors, and the public protection agencies. Probably all three.

I think too many state medical boards, despite their clear duty to protect the public, still believe their first responsibility is to rehabilitate impaired physicians and to protect them from the public's prying eyes. We've seen the definition of "impaired" expanded to cover doctors who may be drunk on the job, strung out on drugs, mentally ill or habitual sex offenders.

I'm not saying it's not important for doctors who suffer from emotional problems or drug or alcohol addiction to receive appropriate treatment, but I do think this must be balanced with the state's responsibility to protect the public from doctors who are not able to deliver good medical care. Some states show a dangerous pattern of letting chemically dependent doctors return to practice after numerous failed attempts at rehabilitation.

L et me read you some 1991 statistics that deal with serious disciplinary actions by state medical licensing boards. Now remember, on average sanctions approach ten per 1,000 doctors.

Who is best and who is worst? Alaska with 18.02 is best, closely followed by Oklahoma with 17.47 and Iowa with 11.63. The most ineffectual states are Rhode Island and South Dakota, who are tied with no serious actions against physicians. Close to the bottom of the list are New York, Massachusetts and Pennsylvania. New York, with 60,744 physicians, took disciplinary action for serious violations against only 54 doctors. That's .89—less than one—per 1,000 doctors. Again, this means, only fifty-four doctors out of over 60,000 were caught for endangering the lives of patients. Massachusetts found only twenty-two out of 21,475 physicians guilty of some serious misdeed. Pennsylvania censured only twenty-two doctors out of 21,475 for incompetence. These are powerful states that should be doing much better. Of course their response was a predictable, "We obviously have better doctors." The truth is that politically, they can't be aggressive as other states.

H ere in California, the director of the Department of Consumer Affairs requested the California Highway Patrol Bureau of Internal Affairs to conduct an investigation of the Medical

Board of California. You might wonder, why the Highway Patrol? The answer is, the State Attorney General's Office serves as the attorney for the Medical Board and there would be a conflict of interest for that department to investigate itself.

It was alleged that top staffers, nicknamed "The Family" by co-workers, practiced nepotism, slept on the job, and abused government cars, gasoline credit cards, frequent flyer credits and cellular phones. The investigation did indeed discover fraud and abuse on the part of some senior staff members of the Medical Board.

It also found that that Medical Board closed hundreds of complaints without review, knowing they would be shredded after sixty days. They did this in order to reduce their backlog—they thought that the best way to cure the problem of questionable physicians was to cleanse the files. Among other findings were the case of a surgeon who inadvertently ruptured (and repaired) the colon of a patient admitted for the removal of an ovarian cyst. During a subsequent operation needed because of complications, that same surgeon punctured the patient's heart, killing her. That case was closed "with merit," meaning the Board's way of getting out of investigating the case was to claim there was insufficient evidence to warrant further investigation.

A car-accident victim admitted to the emergency room was released with instruction to take Advil for pain. Twelve hours later, the patient died from an untreated laceration to the liver and fractured ribs. That case was also closed "with merit."

And, according to the Highway Patrol investigation, the Board staff closed other cases involving allegations that physicians improperly prescribed narcotics to addicts and administered fatal doses of sedatives to patients.

Governor Wilson made heroic efforts to clean up the mess. He appointed a new executive director, replaced the president of the board and ten of the other twenty members. You can praise the governor's actions, but you can't just trade places and change faces. All of the new people are better than the old ones, but they still have to work through the flawed system.

State boards are slow to act on what they have learned. Only a few of the country's best medical boards, for example Utah,

Georgia and Oregon, attempt to act as sleuths, to seek out bad
physicians before receiving complaints, in order to prevent misconduct and poor care.

In the Canadian province of Ontario, the College of Physicians and Surgeons visits physician's offices and performs ran-
dom audits of their care in order assure that licensed physicians
meet minimal requirements for safe practice. Physicians who fail
to meet those standards, and that's as many as twelve percent
of family doctors and two percent of specialists, must undergo
intensive educational retraining, and in rare cases face disciplinary action. No American state has yet attempted such a far-reach-
ing quality control program. Is that because we think the quality
of our doctors is beyond question?

I'm sure everybody read in the spring of 1992, the case of Dr.
Ivan C. Namihas, an Orange County, California gynecologist,
who made headlines for weeks. The medical board received over
one hundred and forty complaints against him, including many
allegations of sexual abuse and inappropriate or improper medical treatment. He used his position of authority as a physician
and as a gynecologist to invade women's most intimate areas of
personal privacy, solely to carry out sexual exploitation for his
own sexual gratification.

What most people probably don't know about is the length of
time it took the state medical board to finally initiate disciplinary
proceedings against him—twenty years. You heard me right.
Twenty years! Apparently, he'd been molesting patients since
1968. As early as 1972, a doctor who moved into the medical
complex shared by Dr. Namihas was warned by other doctors in
the building not to refer patients to him. In 1975, the Orange
County Medical Association had a moment of courage and notified the State Medical Board that three local physicians had received complaints about Dr. Namihas, but no investigation was
started. The Medical Board received another complaint about
him in 1982 and another one in 1987. Still, no investigation was
initiated because the bureaucrats thought the evidence was insuf-

ficient. In 1990 another complaint was received and the light bulb switched on in some incompetent bureaucrat's mind.

Unfortunately, the Board routinely purges its case files if the case is not acted upon for five years. Fortunately a senior investigator had had a strong gut feeling and kept a copy of the file. Two more complaints were received. Finally the story hit the newspapers—the *Orange County Register* did a very credible reporting job—which resulted in one hundred additional complaints regarding sexual abuse by Dr. Namihas.

Wait until you hear this: until March of 1992, the Orange County Medical Association continued to refer patients to Dr. Namihas, even though they were aware of the questions surrounding him. Incredible! Dr. Namihas served on the OCMA committee that checks doctors' credentials for the peer-review process that is intended to weed out bad doctors and prevent them from using the medical society's name to enhance their reputations.

Why didn't the local medical society act against Dr. Namihas? "We have no authority other than to report complaints to the state medical board," was the position of the organization's president. The medical society bemoans the fact that "the public expects us to clean house, but we have no legal right to do it. If we have a bad apple in our midst, we have considerable trouble getting him out of our organization." (Also, the society tosses out complaints after two years regardless of the seriousness of the complaint.)

I wonder, why didn't individual doctors pursue the charges of sexual abuse of their patients? I suppose, some doctors might say, if they had pursued Dr. Namihas more vigorously he would have sued them. Or if they had reported him, they may have been viewed as snitches and cast out of the lucrative referral loop. If they had challenged him, they might have lost their lucrative positions at a hospital where Dr. Namihas was a major shareholder.

One hospital-based physician said, "This is the whole basis for the conspiracy of silence you hear about. He was a member of the board of directors who controlled the hospital-based ancillary service contracts like radiology and the clinical laboratory. There were ten guys waiting to grab my spot. Sure we knew he was a bastard. Why do you think we wouldn't let him be partners or rent space in our office building? We all earned big money investing in the hospital, but we didn't want him too close to home." Another doctor said, "I couldn't do anything because I was gagged by the confidentiality rules that surround hospital disciplinary actions. The man had been called before the medical staff's executive committee to answer charges of molesting patients and nurses."

Through all of this, Dr. Namihas continued to practice at the hospital, and women continued to be molested. Finally, the California Medical Board revoked Dr. Namihas's license. He has since disappeared from sight. Is he doing his thing in another state? I would be surprised to find that out. Is he doing it in another country? That wouldn't surprise me. Did he get away with his crime? He sure did.

D isciplinary action by the state medical board can take three to four years, and then board actions are automatically stayed pending appeal, which permits an offending physician to continue to practice. I read where one Superior Court judge called the board partially responsible for the deaths of eight newborns and a fetus killed by one Los Angeles doctor because they had failed to revoke the doctor's license despite evidence of malpractice.

N o one can argue that questionable doctors can still cross state borders and start right where they left off. There's the case of an Oregon family practitioner who surrendered his Oregon license during a disciplinary investigation and simply moved into California. In fact, during a 1990 hearing of the Oregon Board of Medical Examiners, it was reported that five disciplined doctors were practicing in neighboring states; one of them had been disciplined for incompetence.

T he worst doctors probably work for the federal government. All that is required is to have a medical license from any state government, it doesn't have to be in the state where the doctor is working for the feds. A doctor can have a license from two states, let's say Georgia and California, and his practice comes under question in California. He just ups and leaves before a judgment is rendered, then comes back to the state to work in a VA Hospital, Public Health or Indian Service and he uses the medical license from Georgia. Now do you know why some veterans get such lousy care?

I f we want to correct the problem, the state licensing agencies certainly can clean up their acts by strengthening the medical practice statutes. State boards should be restructured to sever any ties between the board and medical societies. The governor should appoint members to the medical board whose top priority is protecting the public, not providing assistance to the physicians. The state should strip the shield of protection by informing the public of all completed disciplinary actions. State boards should have the authority to impose emergency suspensions pending formal hearings in cases where the doctor poses a potential danger to the public. Finally, boards should accept sanctions imposed by other states, not ignore them.

D octors need a suspension-type process for discipline. With lawyers, you'll get suspended real quick. For instance, if you take one dime out of a trustee account, you run a pretty good risk of being disbarred for life. The first time you'll get ninety days suspension. The second time you'll get maybe a three-year suspension. The third time you're gone for life. It doesn't matter if it's ten cents. You're gone. But in the medical profession, when was the last time you heard of a doctor being disciplined by his peers? Maybe if they get into drugs—maybe. Or maybe if they've gone through a total nervous breakdown, they might not be allowed to continue practicing. You very, very seldom, if ever, find a doctor that's been disciplined for life. I can't remember one.

W e know which doctors to stay away from, but the general public doesn't. I know it's cost prohibitive, but it would sure be nice to have some quality control or consumer group checking up on the doctors in private practice. Hospitals have these controls put upon them by government agencies who come out and inspect them regularly, but the private practice offices don't have anything like that except for OSHA [the Occupational Safety Health Act], and that's only if a patient complains.

Here's a suggestion: There should be an 800 phone number you could call and turn in incompetent or unscrupulous health-care practitioners. This is something not only for the public to use, but for those of us working in the health care. Anonymous tips, just like those available to turn in drug dealers and other criminals. These doctors we know of that are just ripping the system off or endangering patients, we need some type of phone number to call without risking being blackballed in the business. And then, we need an agency that goes in there and verifies the complaint. At worst, it would be an inconvenience to the wrongly accused doctor. At best, it would ensure the safety of patients and help weed out the bad guys.

I was in a position to turn in an individual that was using fraud-ulent advertising, but the only recourse I had was through the state board. The state board is not interested in listening to pro-fessional gripes. They're really a consumer group. They will hear the complaint at a later date, if they have time.

Of course you wouldn't want a health care *Gestapo*, but there needs to be some means where we have recourse when we feel the public is being adversely affected.

I'd like to see the public be encouraged to file complaints re-garding acts of incompetence or inappropriate behavior. Not just let their insurance company handle it.

And I'd like to see the states require periodic recertification for competence. If we are required to renew our driver's license with an examination, why can't a physician be required to take a test every five or ten years. I mean, things are changing so fast in medicine, almost moment to moment, it would force them to keep current.

I s the American Medical Association the most powerful union in the world that protects incompetent physicians from disciplinary action. No. The fault really lies with the state governmental agencies responsible for licensing physicians. I don't think that most people realize that the AMA is only a powerful doctors' political lobby and educational institution. It has absolutely no control over the licensing or disciplining of physicians.

T here have been some realistic and doable suggestions made to correct the disciplinary system for physicians. It's been recommended that the federal government provide the states with grants-in-aid to establish enforceable standards and investigative staffs. Another suggestion is that the Medicare Peer Review Organizations, which don't really discipline incompetent physicians, should become more aggressive by hiring investigators and legal advisers.

It's also been suggested that the information contained in the National Practitioner Data Bank be opened to the public; at present it's limited to hospitals and state agencies. Others want the Drug Enforcement Administration to release a monthly list of all practitioners whose controlled substance prescription licenses have been revoked, restricted or denied. That list should then be widely distributed to pharmacies, and state pharmacy and medical boards. Then the general public should be notified by publication of the names of the physicians sanctioned, and in addition every pharmacy should post in a conspicuous place the names of all physicians who have been disciplined by a regulatory agency.

Hospitals should be mandated to post in appropriate public locations official disciplinary actions against all physicians in their community, and every patient being treated on an outpatient or inpatient basis should be able to review the lists of disciplinary actions. I think a very significant suggestion is that all physicians must be periodically recertified for competency.

D octors tend to be protected because they're next to god. And the AMA and the local medical societies are very powerful. They have not allowed the doctors' licensing program to come under consumer scrutiny. No one can scrutinize a doctor's ability except another doctor, because there's none of us stupid lay people who can understand what it takes to be a doctor. That's bullshit!

I know how doctors work, I've been around them for forty years. There are some beautiful ones. There are some unscrupulous ones. And most of them are just plain guys and gals. They're smarter than the rest of us on an IQ level, no doubt about that, but there's nothing mysterious about them. But they are so brainwashed going through medical school and residency as to their god-like ability, that many of them believe it. That's no bull. Not all of them, most of them are good people, but there are a lot of [expletive deleted] out there that are doctors.

It would probably be an excellent idea to bring the medical licensing board under the department of consumer affairs, and to make sure that not just one lay person sits in judgment on the ones that have screwed up. That would help.

Let's take a look at what happened to the legal profession in the last three or four years. There is a legislative attempt to really take control of the legal profession and to dictate punishment, supervision, and licensing. When I came into the profession in 1975, we were virtually autonomous, much like the doctors are today. That's not so anymore. On the State Board of Governors, I believe there's twelve lawyer-governors and five lay persons. The lay persons are appointed by the governor and the State Senate and the State Assembly. That's brought a different attitude . . . it's not a good ol' boy club by a long shot anymore, it's not business as usual. We've got people in there agitating and representing the lay person. There is disciplinary action for any attorney who messes up, there's a whole court system within the State Bar to investigate, review, listen to the evidence, and suspend—either temporarily or permanently.

Now, the legal profession is much more tightly regulated by the lay people and consumer industry than the doctors' lobby ever conceived that they might be, but lawyers have been made out to be the bad guys so they can get those kind of rules against us. Until doctors have that element of consumer scrutiny, they'll be autonomous and free to police their members as they see fit, and that can mean cover up any indiscretions or unscrupulous acts and hope they go away.

5

GETTING DOWN TO THE
BUSINESS OF MEDICINE

If we could apply a slogan to the evolution of medicine during the last half of this century, it would be, "Business is the Best Medicine." And "MD" would stand for "Making Dollars."

Doctors in private practice are entrepreneurs who encounter the range of problems and temptations faced by small business owners everywhere. However, the nature of a doctor's enterprise affects the lives of millions in ways that cannot be compared to other enterprises and doctors must be held to higher standards of business practice. Most physicians by far strive to meet those standards, but those who choose not to can easily take advantage of the system and the vast amounts of money flowing through it.

What's the primary concern in health care now? Money. It's always money. How can you take care of the patient for the least amount of dollars? It's just that now the money has shifted from the doctors to the insurance providers.

We're here to serve the patient. That's my opinion, but that's an individual's choice. I am irked when I hear of colleagues who come in on a Saturday because a patient is having an emergency and they charge them a couple hundred dollars just to open the door because they're ticked off because they're taken away from their families. They're supposed to handle problems. It may interfere with family time, but that's the nature of the profession.

I saw a physician's assistant, and then when the bill came, it had a doctor's name on it that I had never seen. I got charged the doctor's rate, because the doctor ordered the medication. A PA saw me and diagnosed me and gave it to the doctor and he put his name to it without seeing me, and I still got charged the higher fee. Is that what they mean by cost-effective medicine?

It's unfortunate that it is a business. People are in it to make money. It's unfortunate that so much time needs to be spent on running a business. The sheer effort of running a business and all that it entails, takes away so much time from what you want to do, which is just see patients and have the energy to help them. It's not an unethical thing, but it's an unfortunate thing. It's an unfortunate way that it's got turned around in our society which makes less and less people want to go into health care because of the labor of business and the hours that takes.

It's not uncommon for doctors to see too many patients in a period of time. If you take those numbers and divide it by the time, you see how time pressured they are, but dollars roll out because of that. You can be fooled by the argument, well these people need to see somebody, so you can't turn anybody away. But it doesn't seem like they're always being realistic.

Before we ask what's wrong with the patient, it's, "Do you have insurance? What kind? Do you have any cash?" They answer, "Well, we have seven thousand." "That will get you a couple days." Or it's, "No insurance? Sell your house and come back tomorrow."

It is a business. It's a business that's being yanked from more than one direction. It's a unique situation because you have what's right, which is taking care of the patient. It is also satisfying what a physician wants, which usually is good for the patient but not good from a financial standpoint a lot of times. And then you have administration. So you have three different pulls on the people who are actually taking care of the patients day after day.

Physicians have always been difficult to deal with. That's part of their training. They have some unrealistic expectations that you usually have to dance around and keep them happy because they're the ones who bring the patients to the hospital. But at the same time you do that you have a financial bottom line that administration keeps reminding you of. And if you don't do that, they'll fire you if you're in a management position. And then you have the all-important question of, who are you really there to take care of?

S ome changes in the type of individual who enters nursing are occurring. More men are coming in as a career change. They see it as being able to earn a higher wage. We do have people coming in who have a BS in another area, and they got out there and they couldn't get a job and somebody convinced them that you can get a job in health care.

When I was young, you took nursing in case you didn't get married, or if your husband died, you had a way to earn a living. I think that has put our profession behind because we've had people enter nursing who were not committed to the profession. A significant number of men who come in for the RN and BS degree are using it as a stepping stone to anesthesia or nurse anesthesiologist. They're not really committed to the profession. They see it as a quick way to a bigger income. Right now, nurses start at $15 or $16 an hour, some places it's eighteen. It's not a bad starting wage. I know some of the health educators are thinking, boy, I think I'll look at nursing.

M aybe it's when they see other doctors making seven figures, they start to be enticed by it. Then the focus becomes, I'm just going to use my medical degree as a vehicle to become financially independent. That's OK. I look at doctors like entrepreneurs. They're self-employed business people. I think they deserve to make a good salary. I'm not mad at doctors because they make a lot of money. I'm disgusted at the means that some of these guys use to get it.

I want to believe that physicians go into the field because they have a desire to be helpful. And additionally, they know that they are going to be respected in our communities and country, and that they're going to get a good salary.

But I don't know that that's the primary motivation. I think a lot of it has to do with respect. Physicians are very respected in our country, in our culture. When I was a nurse in a hospital I knew a lot of the young physicians who went into the best paying specialties for that very reason. But I don't know if that was most of them. I think there's still altruism as a reason to go into medicine. I certainly hope so, because they're going to get disappointed when they find out that it's really a people business and if you're not in it for the people, it's not a happy life.

For the guys who get through medical school, it's a tough row to hoe. But once they get that degree and they're out, they've got bankers lined up to finance them all the money they want. They know damn well they're going to make easily two, three, four hundred thousand the first or second year. The ones that don't, there's a few that are dedicated and go to Indian reservations or an HMO, but they're probably in the minority.

I don't have a financial investment in the system like some other people do. I don't have a $250,000 education that I have to repay a loan on. I didn't plan that kind of future for me, so it's not a hardship, but I know a lot of people are going to be economically hurt. I just hope that there's enough people out there that went into it for more than just monetary reasons.

Why do you think all these people are in the medical business? To make money! I know a physician who started a clinic, then he said, "Hey, this is working pretty good. I'll build a second clinic, and a third clinic." The guy hasn't practiced medicine in the last five or six years. He's got this huge corporation that he's running and he's making money.

It's obviously a deep dilemma. The doctors go through an evolution process, so does their staff. A young kid comes out of medical school, he's brilliant. After ten or twelve years of school, all of a sudden, he figures the world owes him a living, so they get into the business. It's the money they want.

Some of my best friends, and some of the most reputable doctors in California, they're really neat guys. But they'll make six, seven, eight thousand dollars a day, which is an unholy amount of money, and that's net to them. These are fellows that I've known for twenty or thirty years, and they all say, "Yeah, but I've earned it. You should have seen how I went through medical school and almost starved to death."

I think maybe two percent, three percent are real dedicated saintly type of guys that are workaholics—and they die early. But the average doctors, they'll work hard at the beginning, they'll get their practice going fast, and soon they're making a lot of money. But it's an insatiable thing. There's no such thing as enough money.

I used to be a surgical tech for a local gynecologist here in town. Originally I worked at the hospital, but this doctor gave me an offer I couldn't refuse—lots of money, the best pay I ever had in fact, without working nights, weekends or holidays.

He had three abortion rooms in the clinic, and I just followed him from one room to another. The girls were always prepared and waiting for us. It took about fifteen minutes for each. The doctor uses a vacuum curette—fairly reliable and fast. He can evacuate the uterus in no time for $300 without any responsibility for counseling or follow-up. It's really kind of a boring job, but he sure makes the money. The business office manager once told me he takes home over $1,750,000 a year. Can you believe it? One

million seven hundred and fifty thousand dollars! Now there's a
guy who's definitely pro-choice.

My wife's grandfather was the founder of a large hospital
here. Before he died, when he wound up in bed on his
back, there were two things he told me that I'll never forget. He
said of his golden years: "I worked all my life to make a whole
bunch of gold and the last two years they took all my gold away.
These fucking doctors are only in it for the money." That's what
he said after dealing with the doctors for all his life, his golden
years were when they took all his gold. And the last thing he said
was, "You know, if you stay with the same doctor long enough,
he'll kill you."

A doctor will ask me, "How many mammograms do I have to
do a day to pay for this thing?" Some of my clients, where
there's seven or eight doctors, there's no problem in funneling
the number of patients through to fit that need.

Doctors have hurt themselves because they're not a normal
business. They're used to making five hundred to 1,000 percent on their goods. If it costs them a dollar, they want five dollars
back on it.

They come up with their pricing and they justify it in a million
different ways. Yes, they do have malpractice to worry about, but
the doctors I sell equipment to usually want a return back on their
purchase in less than a year. That's on a $15,000 or $20,000 investment. He wants all his money out of it in six to ten months.
That's what doctors I sell to are telling me.

Normal businesses, when they buy a piece of equipment,
they're looking at two or three years or longer to get all their
money back. The doctors are saying, "No, no. I want it back in
six months." In the past, they've been able to do it, and then it's
just a cash register.

Doctors have cut their nose off to spite their face—health care
is getting into the politicians' hands now. In the past, the mark

ups doctors have been getting have been ridiculous. We've all known that in the business. The nurses know it, the staffs know it, the suppliers know it. The only people that didn't know was the general public. Now the politicians know and want a piece of it, and the doctors are sitting there going, "Poor, poor me." Give me a break.

Yesterday, I was talking to a doctor who bought some equipment from me a year or so ago. I tried to tell him at the time it was inappropriate for his practice, but he didn't want to listen. Now he wants to get a better system because he knows that he's getting poor results. Remember, he's still making the same amount of money, whether he has a new one or keeps the one he's got. Reimbursement to him is the same.

So I called him yesterday and said, "Here's a product you can get. I'll knock down the price twenty-five hundred bucks." He said, "How much do I get off for my trade-in?" I said, "That includes your trade-in. Twenty-five hundred dollars off the new product, plus you give me your old unit." He screamed. "Whoa! What are you saying? It's going to cost me six thousand dollars to upgrade to a new system?" I said, "Yeah, it's a nine thousand dollar unit." Again, he screams. "Oh, no way! I'm not going to pay six thousand dollars. If you can do it for about two thousand dollars, I'll consider it." I said, "Thank you. I've got to go. I can't help you."

A lot of doctors are now employees. I have a big group that I sell to that have a bunch of freestanding clinics. It's like a small HMO. The doctors used to have contracts of thirty percent of gross. Well, thirty percent of gross is a hell of a lot of money, but when you take into consideration that people don't pay their bills and insurance reimbursements are going lower and lower, and these guys are still getting thirty percent of the gross, it was only a matter of time before they had to shut their doors.

So this group told the doctors, "We're putting you on contract. You will become an employee and we'll pay you so many dollars a year and that's it. Take it or leave it." And the doctors took it.

D octors have been living the high life for so long. They have been bringing in so much money. But doctors are not very good business people, first of all, no matter what they think. They spend. They have a tendency to spend their money. Spend, spend, spend. It's been, "Oh, yeah, no big deal. We're doctors. There's plenty more money where that came from."

Well, all of a sudden the balloon has popped for the doctors and their reimbursements are going down. The patients are shifting into PPOs and HMOs. All of a sudden doctors are saying, "Wait a minute. What happened to half of my patient load?" Then they're asking, "Who's going to pay the mortgage on my three vacation homes? Who's going to pay the insurance on my luxury cars? Who's going to pay for the lifestyle that I've grown accustomed to? That I deserve!"

I t's OK to do an angiogram that costs $2,500 if the patient needs it, but now you've got Magnetic Resonance, you've got Computerized Tomography ultrasound—you've got other modalities that can assess the patient's condition better than just a typical blood work-up. The problem is that in many cases, they'll have all of them done. They'll have the ultrasound, CT, the MRI, and then go and have the angio, too. Some doctors get used to relying on everything—and then abusing everything. They end up detrimentally affecting the costs to the patient.

Ideally, they'll start off with a noninvasive study. You want to stop wherever you can stop with the least amount of invasion and least amount of dollars.

Dollars is what it boils down to. If they're going to give you $6 to do the study and it's going to cost you $10 after you've gone through three tests to find the positive, you're going to want to stop at the first indication that it's negative.

M edicaid is so difficult. The reimbursement is so hard. On a $40 office visit, you get $11 reimbursement which doesn't even pay for your office staff to prepare the papers to get reimbursed. It really turns into charity work.

M edicaid tells you they're going to pay $10 a chem panel. If it's got more than seven tests on it that are part of the SMAC panel, they're going to pay you $13 whether you run seven or twenty. If you run three to five, they'll pay you $7. So they set the prices, and you can bill anything that you want, they won't pay you. Everybody sends them the full bill, and they just kind of laugh at you and send you your twelve bucks or whatever. When they're ready to.

That's a big problem for labs, delayed payments from the government. It's put a lot of guys out of business. The bureaucracy, the slow payback. Being in the hospital business, as you know, they have some high school kid reviewing the thing and rejecting your claim. Meanwhile you still have to pay your employees, the reagents to do the test, and the time and everything else involved. They rejected you because you didn't dot an "i" or some very insignificant thing. You wonder if that's the way the government's working to keep the cashflow positive.

I can't tell you what reimbursement rates are. I know that my hospital customers keep complaining because reimbursements keep going down and down and down and down. Medicare and Medicaid don't pay very well, and they have to take in so many indigent patients that don't pay at all. So some of these clinics I deal with don't take anything unless it's cash or good insurance. They get top dollar for everything they do.

W hen I first started, money was easy. The laboratory, instead of being a cost center, was a revenue center. That meant that raises came automatically. That meant that they were adding staff once they justified it, regardless of how they justified it. If there was some benefit out of it, they'd hire somebody. It was a geometrically growing type of situation.

So why did these ancillary areas go from being revenue to cost centers? Reimbursement. It used to be they just increased their prices if they wanted to grow. At that time insurance companies were just paying what came through. They paid ninety percent of everything, or eighty percent of everything. It was really rather simple. There wasn't competition. There were enough people out there to fill the beds. People didn't shop for health care. Therefore, they could just arbitrarily raise their prices.

Then all of a sudden DRGs came and everything changed. [DRGs were developed by Medicare to calculate how much certain medical procedures should cost; and therefore, how much the health-care provider would be reimbursed.] I worked in Orange County at the time; hard times hit Orange County a lot sooner than most places, probably seven, eight, nine years ago. Maybe even ten years ago. People really had to look at the bottom line, at reimbursement. From that standpoint, health care became a business at a certain level in a hospital. Especially the support services. Nursing to a certain degree. Physicians, not at all. Administration, a little bit. But the support services were strongly hit, so there were cutbacks. That was a very difficult time, especially for hospitals because their services were very poor then.

Now, what we're seeing is, not only did they start looking at it as a business, but they started looking at it the way the Japanese looked at business. And this is the big push now—I'd like to see more of it—quality improvement. In other words, you want to be in competition with other neighborhood hospitals. This is against the Clinton plan. The patient, your doctor, they're your customer. You don't go into a hospital and become a number.

So business has gone full circle. It was not a business; it was just uninhibited growth, a creature that was just growing geometrically, then DRGs hit, that became a business, scrutinizing expenses, both capital and for employment. Now they're looking at it as being a customer-oriented type of a business. So they're kind of going full circle again, and that means sometimes you're going to have to hire extra people to do the right thing.

Marketing drugs directly to the consumer is a new trend. Patients should not be going into doctor's offices saying, "I want this drug." The scenario should be, the physician makes the diagnosis and then consults with the pharmacist to determine which medication is proper to use in which situation. Under no circumstances should the patient be coming in with an ad from *Time* magazine saying, "I want to try this."

There's a new headache medication out on the market. One injection is $18, and the doctor sells it for $75. Seventy-five dollars. I can't believe they're charging that much money. But if someone has a migraine, they're going to pay it.

Prepackaged meds that are being sold through the "Doc-in-the-box" clinics is another area of gouging the public. For instance, if you take your daughter in, say she's sick on a Saturday, you're there and they say, "If you want to buy this prepackaged amoxycillan for her today, you can buy it from us." They're turning around and being a drug store and making a big profit on it. I know what they pay, I sell it to them. They're doubling and tripling their money on the medications. They're making lots of money at the expense of a "captive" patient.

Access to pharmaceuticals is one thing that really does need to be looked at more closely. I sell pharmaceuticals. I have one account out in a remote area, and they have a patient that comes in every week for chemotherapy. He has no insurance. I'm talking zero. But because he has cancer, he has to have that drug. I know what it costs and I know what it sells for, and it's ridiculous. It costs $300 for the company I work for, and the cost to the doctor is $650. In our pharmaceuticals, well, in some of our other items I can price them the way I want them, but my company has to get $650. Then the doctor adds probably twenty-five percent on top of that. That brings it up to over $800 for each injection. And this man has to pay for that out of his pocket. He's not a wealthy man, but if he wants to stay alive, he'll pay it.

It's just not right. If a patient is sick and dying and doesn't have the money to pay for it, we should have something available for these people. Give it to them at cost at the very least. If a drug company did that and cut out the middlemen, it wouldn't put anybody in the poor house, and it would sure make a difference for those people in need.

D rug companies will tell you out of one side of the mouth that they spent $16 billion in research and development last year, but not tell you that they spent ten percent more than that on advertising. Wait a minute! If they have these tax breaks to help them with their cost of research (by manufacturing their drugs in Puerto Rico for example) and they're spending more money on advertising than they spend on research, what are we subsidizing, the research or the advertising?

T here's a contrast agent used in MRI. It was the first one that came out. They had a lock on the market for about five years. List price on ten bottles of that stuff, a 20cc bottle, was $2,180. So what's that, $218 a bottle? That's ten bucks a cc. Of course the manufacturer is claiming that they had to put a lot of money into research and development for that product. But how long does it take to pay back R&D?

Now two other companies have come out with the same product, but they're all priced the same. No one wanted to start a price war here. It's not in their best interests. And of course that cost gets passed on to the public.

There's another. Non-ionic contrast material. It has no iodine in it, you have a lot less reactions. When that first came out, the stuff was prohibitively expensive, and it still is very, very expensive. Here's the scenario: if you're a hospital, and you can't afford to buy that stuff and you used iodinated contrast material and someone dies because of an adverse allergic reaction, and you knew full well that other contrast material was out there, you'll be litigated in the next month. And you'll lose because there was something that was better for the patient but you didn't use it. It doesn't matter if you couldn't afford to.

You can't go to the patient and say, "Which one do you want to use? This one costs a hundred dollars. This one costs twenty dollars." Of course the patient is going to say the hundred dollar one. So you're damned if you do and damned if you don't.

I f you look at the largest pharmaceutical companies, pharmaceuticals are just one part of their makeup. Making a profit, that's the reason they're in the pharmaceutical business, they're in it to make money. If you look at the industry world-wide, American pharmaceuticals are the leaders. I think Japan has one company that competes with us, only one.

To me, this means that we must be doing something right. Because they have capital to reinvest in research, a researcher can work for forty years and not come up with a single good drug, but they'll still give him a paycheck every Friday. How many other industries still do that? The reason why pharmaceutical companies do, is that when someone does discover a new drug, they make their money back.

We're leaders in pharmaceutical technology, and if the government tries to take away the profit, these companies will simply move their resources into another area and we'll be left with an industry that stagnates.

I n the area that I compete in, the doctors look at me like your Chevrolet dealer. They'll go to one dealer and want to buy a Caprice Classic and the guy will give them a price and they'll say, "To hell with that." Then they'll go over to another dealer and get a price, and then another dealer. They really want to get the best price. They don't care how long you've been in business. They don't care that you're going to be around when they run into problems with the state inspectors and all that sort of stuff. All they want is the best deal that they can find.

The manufacturer is the only one who wins. If there's three or four people all selling the same product and they're cutting each other's throats, the manufacturer still gets the order. And of course these doctors that buy the machines, they're still going to charge whatever they're going to charge.

T hings are really changing in medical supplies, especially with all the HMOs popping up everywhere. It used to be a rep like me would pull up to the one little doctors' office on the corner, Dr. Jones and Dr. Smith, and write an order. Those guys now are dropping like flies and going in with larger groups. When they do, suddenly I have to be able to offer hospital pricing on supplies or I lose the business. In most cases, our pricing structure doesn't allow me to do that. I work for a small supplier. Some of our pricing is good and some of it isn't.

My biggest facility has thirty-two doctors who left a well-known clinic about two years ago and started their own group. I set them all up, along with several satellite offices they've got. But I'm in there right now only because of my level of service. That's it, because they can get far better pricing from the hospital vendors. I won't be surprised when they finally make that decision to go for the lowest price. It all happens so fast that you can't even keep up with it. Blink your eyes and. . . .

I know at that hospital, they recruited a radiologist out of the East someplace. He was a pediatric radiologist or some crazy thing like that. While they were negotiating with him, the guy said, "No, I like it here at this hospital because they just bought me this special equipment that I wanted." The doctor that was recruiting said, "Not a problem. You come join the group and we'll clone that one. We'll get you the identical thing." They called up the manufacturer's rep and asked for the identical machine, and about a week later he came with a quote of well over a million.

The point I'm trying to make is they could have gone with another manufacturer and got the same identically performing unit, maybe the buttons are in a different place, but is as good if not better a machine at a price that wasn't quite as steep. But they wanted the business that doctor could bring in so they were willing to give him what he wanted.

The last time I had any dealings with a certain hospital, they were building a couple of outpatient centers. They were going to buy two mammography machines plus a CT for each one. These were nice places.

I made my proposal, and at that time it was state-of-the-art equipment, nothing to be ashamed of. They ended up buying from another dealer. But the equipment they bought was almost twice as expensive as my machine. The argument was, "If it costs half as much, obviously it's only half as good."

I happened to be at a trade show, and there was one of the vice presidents from that hospital that was there recruiting. I had a machine on display and she came over and said, "I don't know anything about radiology, but this is kind of a neat machine." So I showed it to her, and she said, "You know, I bet our hospital could use a couple of these." So I told her my story, and she was absolutely flabbergasted that they wouldn't even consider it because it didn't cost enough.

I was talking to a guy the other day who's buying a new CAT scanner for his hospital . . . a few years ago he bought a CAT scanner. That's the problem with where technology is headed. By the time you buy something and get it installed, they come out with something else and you either need to upgrade or get rid of it, or use what you have until you can justify buying a new one.

He said he bought the best CAT scanner he could buy with all the options, and he paid over $1,000,000 for this CAT scanner. And now he's looking to either upgrade the unit or buy a new one, and his unit is only three or four years old, but he feels his hospital has to keep up with state-of-the-art to hang on to their share of the market.

The used equipment business has picked up and the service business has too. If you're in the service business right now, you're one of the few areas of health care that are making a good profit. Every time something breaks, instead of going out and replacing it, doctors and hospitals are keeping the old technology, keeping the old horse running. They're going to do with the old nag rather than replace it with a new car. If you're in the service business, you're happy.

Rising costs are also a result of a throwaway mentality that we have. Nothing is used more than once. Everything is disposable. There's so much waste now, it makes me sick. We used to autoclave everything, but you see you can't anymore, because it may create questions or doubts regarding sterilizing techniques and if you get sued, you'll lose. Patients are going to get infections anyway, but if they decide to sue you, and the lawyers make a point out of the fact that you reused supplies, you'll lose the case.

I t's scary for everybody involved. You can get a catastrophic illness and it'll wipe out your life savings in a matter of a couple of weeks. My father just had double bypass surgery back East, and the bill so far is $50,000 and the bills are still coming.

What makes an aspirin $5? What makes a Band-Aid $2? The catheters we use in angio, why do they cost us $1,000 each and we use them once only? A thousand bucks, we use them on somebody and in the trash it goes.

A chief executive officer of one of the third-party insurance intermediaries goes around the country now, telling us that we're going to have to just get used to getting by with less money, that we're getting paid too much. I am damned sick and tired of listening to a man who makes twenty times what I make in a year tell me the problem is I'm making too much money. These CEOs make fabulous amounts of money, and they don't consider themselves to be part of the problem as far as pricing?

E very hospital that participates in the Medicare program is subject to a field audit by accountants representing the US government. Reviewing all the accounting records of a hospital is a tedious job that can sometimes take months to complete. Usually, they discover paybacks, at least enough to cover the accounting exercise. It's very, very rare for them to find that Medicare has underpaid on claims. In this particular hospital we're talking about, our people feared we were in deep trouble even before the auditors arrived.

As you know, in our state, prostitution is legal. Auditors away from home for long periods are like sailors at sea on long voyages. The hospital controller understood that. He also knew that "problems" were bound to be found by unfriendly and bored auditors, so he took them to one of our famous brothels. When it came time to pay, the controller whipped out the official hospital credit card. No questions were asked by the madam.

Well, the audit concluded without incident, and the exit conference held with all the bigwigs present was one of praise and fond remembrances. Much to the surprise of the hospital staff, the auditors announced we were to receive additional reimbursement! After the visitors left the room, the hospital's vice president for finance was congratulated profusely by his superiors who recognized that the potential for major financial penalties had vaporized.

Next month, a group of us from accounts payable visited the hospital's CEO. Our spokesperson said, "Should we pay this invoice? There's a major charge by our boss for 'services' at that place up the road." Then she said something like, "We all find the expense insulting. And it's fraudulent. What are you going to do about it?"

Apparently, within hours, the vice president for finance was summoned to the CEO's office. Expecting no problems, he entered without hesitation. The CEO blew his stack. "Why the hell didn't you pay cash or ask me for my credit card? The whole office is in an uproar and they want your head on a platter. And you know what, they're going to get it. I have decided to accept your resignation because you're starting a private consulting business. Your first contract will be with us for six months, so clean your office out as fast as you can."

6

MILKING THE SYSTEM

The potential for fraud and abuse in the medical system is staggering. The problems range from unnecessary $50,000 surgeries to billing for tests the lab is running for free. Fraud can be found at the level of the individual practitioner and that of the corporate provider—and everywhere in between. All told, the total dollar amount of medical-related fraud is astonishing. Some estimates indicate that it may exceed one tenth of all health-care expenditures. Any single chapter can merely highlight a few aspects of the problem, so we chose to concentrate on the potential for fraud in laboratory work, because its technical nature almost precludes patient understanding of the process.

From $50 billion to $90 billion of our money disappears every year in the nation's biggest unchecked scandal, which is medical fraud. It's been described as an orgy of economic crime. As the country's health-care bill hovers around $900 billion annually, it has become an open target for a wily and professional group of criminals. The efficiency marvels of the modern electronic age have further confused the audit trail that paper used to leave. Health-care fraud is many times greater than the scandalous savings and loan debacle, but like that disaster, the consumers and businesses are going to pay for it for a long time to come. Unlike the S&L crimes, there hasn't been political or journalistic demands for justice.

There's always been fraud committed by health-care providers, but today's scam artists are more blatant, cunning, ambitious, talented and organized. A former inspector general of the Department of Health and Human Services said, "A welfare queen would have to work mighty hard to steal $100,000, but a health-care provider can burp and steal $100,000."

E thics, unfortunately, is strictly related to whether they're going to sanction you for doing something wrong and you're going to lose something. If you lose your right to practice your craft, that's a big loss. One of the problems we have in health care is that once people are committing abuses, be they misdemeanors or felonies, the fines or the punishments are nothing. You defraud the government for six million bucks on Medicare, they'll give you three months in the county jail. You do a little time, but you're a millionaire. After that you don't have to worry about anything. That's crazy.

You should be stripped of your license to operate. The laws are there. The facts are clear. Everybody understands right and wrong. Again, our goal is to serve the public, not to rip off the public. Everybody understands that and to go ahead and do it anyway and get away with it, I think is a sin.

T he government has not issued a firm estimate of the annual cost of health-care fraud, but inside officials in the various medical industries estimate that fraud totals approximately ten percent of all health-care expenditures. Changing the national delivery system will not deter criminals. They will only find a way to exploit the new system. I think that if we are to provide health care for all of our citizens, we must find a way to dramatically reduce medical fraud.

Are physicians to blame for the fraud and abuse? Some doctors are corrupt, but the majority are completely honest. However, without physicians, medical fraud and abuse would be minimal.

Doctors, whether they like it or not, whether they are involved or merely bystanders, are the skilled players in this game of greed that is costing billions of dollars every year.

From the second world war until the late 1980s, most, if not all of the fraud in medical laboratories was committed by individuals or small groups of scam artists. That's not to say that the extent of the crime was minimal. The "Russians" pulled off a major criminal operation. In the early 1990s two Russian immigrant brothers, Michael and David Smushkevich, filed nearly $1 billion in false claims, of which they received $50 million paid for by Medicare, Medicaid and private insurers. Fifty million! The operation at its peak involved 1,000 phony companies and 400 bank accounts scattered worldwide. The Smushkeviches operated through "rolling labs" in health clubs, shopping malls, retirement homes, mobile home parks, community health fairs and eventually freestanding clinics. They would conduct unnecessary and frequently fake tests on unsuspecting patients who paid nothing while billing insurance companies or the government programs for the full costs. Faking tests is known as the "sink method." You pour the patient's test down the sink's drain and fake the results so that they would justify a diagnosis that would justify payment.

It's amazing how just plain gullible people are for con artists. The rolling lab fraud solicited patients through "boiler room" telemarketing operations. Telephone solicitors would offer comprehensive physical exams with state-of-the-art diagnostic testing. If they could get the patient into one of the clinics, the bill for a two-hour visit would average $7,500. To make this scam work, the con artists would bill, not for preventive tests, but for tests that correlated with falsified illnesses. That way, they had a justified medical necessity which is a prerequisite for insurance payment. Often these tests were performed before the physical examination.

Their fraud was uncovered when a physician employee of a major insurance company was solicited by a telemarketer. Curiosity led the physician to participate. In his case, his own company was billed for almost $8,000, all with a false medical diagnoses on the claims.

It took eight months for authorities to raid the operation. When they finally did, the brothers and their helpers were charged with over 150 counts of mail fraud, money laundering, and racketeering. Of course the Smushkevich brothers pleaded that they were absolutely not guilty.

That's not the end of the story. There were disastrous consequences for the innocent patients. The wild diagnoses ended up in some insurance companies files. You can imagine the patients' frustration and anger when later turned down for insurance for preexisting conditions. It took years to clear most records, and the patients were never compensated for the pain, suffering and fraud they endured.

That kind of fraud didn't end with the Smushkevich brothers. They were, I guess you would say, pioneers in it, but in comparison to the current group of con artists out there, they're amateurs.

When we use the word "mill," those are the ones that are not legitimate medical facilities. Either they're not licensed or they're known as facilities that work up workers compensation claims in order to get paid. In the fraudulent claims, the doctor will see the patient for a few minutes, and then turn around and charge us $1,200 or $1,500 for a consultation that only lasted a few minutes. That's how they make their money. They charge us for a medical/legal examination, and they've never really examined the patient thoroughly, and in some cases never saw the patient at all. Sometimes during a deposition, we'll ask the patient what the doctor looked like. The patient can't say because they were never examined.

I'm aware of what they call the stress-testing mills. The way they work is this. Someone calls your home and says, "I'm doing a survey on health care and medical insurance. My first question is do you have any?" The person will often answer, "Yeah, I've got an eighty/twenty plan and the deductible is a hundred dollars." After a few more questions, they set the bait. "For participating in our survey, we're offering you a full extensive physical at no cost." Of course you're surprised and say somewhat cynically, "At no cost?" And they answer, "Well, no cost to you. We'll just take whatever your insurance pays."

You wouldn't believe how many people buy into this. They'll come into the local clinic and bring their insurance card, and the next thing you know, they've run up $3,000 to $4,000 worth of testing. The mill knows in advance what the insurance company will reimburse for, so there's no doubt whether they'll be reimbursed or not.

And to ensure that they do, they have patient questionnaires. Insurance companies won't pay for diagnostic procedures unless you have a symptom that warrants it, so these questionnaires ask, "Does heart disease run in your family? Do you smoke? Do you have shortness of breath?" All questions intended to find a workable symptom that a patient could check "yes" to. Then boom, they can order the stress test. That's what they're doing. They're milking the system.

I dentifying which medical groups are practicing workers comp fraud is not just based on the number of claims that are handled, it's more just becoming familiar with their reports and reading their reports. Some of them are very blatant computer-generated reports, where some keyboard operator puts it into a computer program and the report is just putting this questionnaire into narrative form. Some are more sophisticated than others. I was sent a demonstration disk for one of these because I'm an MD, and they thought I might be interested in doing some workers comp.

It's very interesting that the doctor gets paid $1,200 for several hours' work, and yet this questionnaire doesn't take any time for the doctor. It will maybe take an hour for some person that's being paid minimum wage. The doctor obviously has to see it, but in some cases it's so fraudulent that the doctor doesn't even see the individual. But for the great majority, the doctor does see the individual for a short period of time, but it's not adequate for them to do an evaluation, what they're getting paid for and what they're supposed to be doing.

For, I'd say nearly thirty years, some suppliers have been treating Medicare like an open checkbook. Crooked suppliers ripoff the government and patients for millions annually by selling overpriced and unnecessary equipment to the elderly.

The classic case is one supplier in Philadelphia who had teenage girls calling Medicare beneficiaries who had responded to a newspaper ad offering a "free Medicare-covered package." The telemarketers would get the elderly person's Social Security number and ask them if they had any physical complaints. If they did, the firm said they could get equipment that would help. Even though Medicare requires a twenty percent copayment, the senior citizen would be told that Medicare would pay one hundred percent for everything. How could teenagers, without any medical training, make diagnoses regarding expensive equipment? They did.

The prescription form for Medicare equipment required a doctor's signature. The firm got legitimate signatures. The forms were already filled out by the company, and if you think the doctors were too busy to notice what they were signing, you are not alone. Then too, sometimes the doctors figured the patients must really feel they need it, and other times their patients pressured them into signing the forms. Or, do you think physician and supplier kickbacks could have been the motive?

In many frauds, the equipment is not only nonessential but outrageously overpriced. For example, foam pads that cost about $30 were sold for $900. One scheme was to ship the equipment from different regions in the US where Medicare allowed higher prices. A seat cushion that Medicare pays $42 for in Tennessee, will be reimbursed at $249 in Pennsylvania. One guess where the scam artist lists the selling location?

National Health Laboratories, an indirect subsidiary of Revlon, Inc., is one of the six largest medical laboratories in the

United States. In December of 1992, National pleaded guilty to charges of submitting false claims to Medicare and other federal health insurance programs and agreed to pay $111.4 million to settle the civil and criminal suits filed by the Department of Justice. The president of the company resigned after also pleading guilty to the same two counts of criminal fraud.

Here is how the scam worked. The most commonly ordered test is an automated chemistry panel that from one small blood specimen can give twenty to twenty-four individual test results in one minute at ten percent of the cost of individually doing the tests. These tests, called SMAC 20 or SMAC 24—SMAC stands for Sequential Multi-Analysis Computer—are highly informative, relatively inexpensive and quickly performed and are probably the most commonly ordered tests by physicians. For lab tests to be paid for by insurance companies and federal programs, the physician must state that the tests are required for diagnosis and treatment; a test must be reasonable and necessary. With SMACs, the medical necessity of only one test is required. The costs of one test or twenty-four automated tests are approximately the same.

National Labs was cute and cunning. They marketed the SMAC chemistry panel as a part of a Health Survey Panel to which they had added two tests not run on a SMAC. National added HDL cholesterol and serum ferritin. If a physician wanted to order the SMAC, he had to also take the two tests for a small additional charge of 65 cents to $1.20. (If the doctor bitched enough, there would be no charge for the extras.) But where National billed the insurers directly, like in the case of Medicare, it charged separately for the extras to the tune of $20 for the cholesterol and $18 for the ferritin. Here's an example of what this means—in 1988, Medicare paid National $500,000 for ferritin tests. In 1990, after the ferritin was added and billed separately, Medicare paid $31,000,000 for ferritin testing.

What else happened to National Health Laboratories? Nothing. They are still permitted to participate in federal Medicare and Medicaid programs. I would venture that their post-penalty profits are enormous.

What irks me the most is that a lab like National, which is one of the largest laboratory networks in the world, defrauded the government for upwards of $100 million and they can still be open. They got fined a lot of money, but hey, they committed fraud and they're still operating.

C LIA law [the Clinical Laboratory Improvement Act] is a set of rules describing acceptable laboratory techniques for carrying out certain tasks—they're trying to set up a standardized protocol which is acceptable and valid throughout the country and throughout each lab, be it the physician's lab, be it the licensed clinical lab, be it the hospital lab, the reference lab, whatever.

There's all kinds of arguments about what the standards should be. Like, should you allow a high school kid to do testing, or should you require a college degree? That's a real controversy because under that set of rules, they're proposing a lot of the work to be done by what most of us consider people that are underqualified. True, you can get them cheaper, but this is all about improving the quality of the testing across the nation.

California, New York, Florida and a few other states have a set of laws governing laboratory personnel as they would for physicians, their education and what they can and cannot do with their training. Some states don't, they have a set of guidelines. So while it's an actual law in some states, it's only recommended in others.

T he training of med techs is very comprehensive. It's a graduate school level of training. The licensed people, if they do things wrong, they're going to lose their license. They're going to lose anywhere from five to ten years of education, whatever they're doing. So there's also the real fear factor in there. If we just conducted our business like it's stated, I don't think there would be anything wrong.

The national requirements allow high school kids to run tests. They've lowered the professional standards and qualifications for the workers, but they've increased the standards of the testing itself in terms of technical requirements. It's like having a race car and taking an experienced driver out and putting in a high school kid to drive the car. Maybe he'll get through, maybe he won't.

Here are two examples of how physician lobbies have managed to dilute the quality standards set by CLIA—of course this benefits the physician's pocketbook. One, personnel standards were modified to allow physicians to be laboratory directors and to fill all personnel categories in moderately complex labs. Two, testing personnel standards were changed drastically to allow physicians to hire those with minimum training. Proficiency testing requirements would be phased in slowly which means nobody was concerned with the accuracy of test results in physician-owned labs. They're basically saying, "Let people be misdiagnosed now because it would be too inconvenient or expensive for the doctor to be accurate."

Anyone who has ever managed a hospital, knows that ninety-five percent of physicians are not competent to supervise medical clinical laboratories. For most physicians, to be a lab director, is like having licensed automobile drivers, without effort and education, be automobile mechanics and safety officers. A license to practice medicine and surgery is certainly not an endorsement to direct a medical lab.

Is it feasible for a doctor to have a lab? It depends on his practice. In purchasing lab equipment for an office, the salesmen come in, they tell them this, they tell them that. These salesmen are usually not health-care professionals. Some of them may be licensed techs, but let's put it this way, what's the salesman's motive? Money. He'll sell you anything he can, anywhere, anytime. There's nothing wrong with that, that's their vocation. But a potential buyer has to remember they're not necessarily going to be selling you the best product or trade you properly. Not necessarily.

So what happens is, the doctors wind up buying instruments that are not cost effective for them. It may not be applicable to their operation because of special retraining required, or in some cases not having appropriate staffing and equipment, so they end up losing money. In that case, no, doctors should not have labs in their office. But if they pick the right tests and the right methodologies, they would make additional income and benefit the patient.

The size of the potential fraud and abuse is related to the number of medical laboratories. Statistics show that. The estimates of the number of labs subject to CLIA '88 range from 180,000 to 250,000. The intermediate assumption, based on estimates of physician-owned labs by the AMA, is 210,000.

Of this number, 7,000 are hospital based, 6,000 are freestanding proprietary labs, 130,000 are physician-owned and 67,000 are in nursing facilities, ambulatory surgical centers, home health agencies, prisons, student health services, family planning clinics and sexually-transmitted disease clinics. Of the doctor labs, 90,000 are primary care physicians and 40,000 are non-primary care physician ownership.

Since 1980, the clinical laboratory market has continued to grow with a fifteen percent annual growth rate, and the physician-owned lab has been the most rapidly expanding segment of the industry. It is estimated that the doctor labs represent fifty percent of all outpatient testing, at higher costs per test and without satisfactory quality control standards.

The federal government estimated that laboratory testing is a $30 billion business. Others estimate, of that total, $7.5 billion is in independent and reference labs, $15 billion in hospitals, and $7.7 billion in physician labs. For the doctors, that would be nearly $57,700 per year. That's not bad for incidental office income. Now can you see why the AMA doesn't want CLIA '88? Sure, some of the resistance is against excessive regulations, but certainly the greed motive can't be discounted.

In a political preemptive strike, the American Medical Association's House of Delegates supported strict guidelines that generally prohibit referrals to medical facilities in which doctors invest but do not practice. Of course a means of circumventing this is provided if the community lacks such alternative sources of testing, a claim that can be made by playing word games.

The Florida Health Care Cost Containment Board analyzed 2,600 state health-care facilities in order to determine how many joint ventures were owned by physicians and medical groups. At least forty percent of physicians in Florida were involved in joint ventures where they can refer patients. This is clearly a conflict of interest and potential for fraud and abuse. There was no question that overutilization occurred in Florida joint ventures. The number of tests per patient in doctor-owned labs was 3.3 compared with 1.7 in noninvested labs. The average charge in doctor-owned labs was $43 per patient versus $20 at other labs.

I really don't think there's anything inherently evil in joint ventures. They're used to develop services that don't exist or to enhance the ability to deliver services. Those needs will still be present if the joint venture ceases to be. But the main question is how can the ownership formula be developed to prevent the known potential for fraud and abuses.

The IRS has begun an active campaign against certain hospital-physician joint ventures that could threaten the tax exempt status of some not-for-profit hospitals. These joint ventures involved deals in which hospitals sold "net revenue streams" from outpatient surgical centers and other diagnostic and therapy units.

Here's how that deal worked. Under the guise of improving efficiency, hospitals sold the profits from a department for a fixed period of time and future revenues. The doctors do well since the price that they pay for future net revenues is based on the department's past performance. The doctors benefit directly from the earnings increases on the patient referrals that they are likely to increase. These deals were designed to retain physicians, undermine competition, and increase referrals. Gaining a larger portion of the market share is a legitimate business goal, but the creativity of some joint ventures destroy the health-care ethics system.

A fter seeing your doctor in his office, it's so convenient to pick up your prescription at the first-floor pharmacy as you leave the building. The office nurse is so thoughtful and considerate she even offers to call the prescription downstairs so it'll be waiting for you when you get off the elevator. No wasted time. And when you're not feeling well, who needs the aggravation of going to another pharmacy?

What the patient doesn't know is that the doctor, if he is an owner of the building, gets a cut of the profit on your prescription. It's done legally, or at least without any direct evidence. You see, the pharmacist who leases space in the medical building has to put cash up front before the lease is signed. The doctor owners, rather than report this as income, apply it to the completion of their own offices and take a business tax deduction for it. The lease for the pharmacy provides for a percentage of the gross sales to the doctors who own the building. What's happening is that some of the money you're paying to the pharmacy is going directly back to the doctor.

And meanwhile, you're thanking him for making it so convenient.

K ickbacks. Let me just go into the rationale about them briefly. What they're trying to do is induce needless ordering of lab tests. That's generally the outcome of it—encouraging physicians to order tests that are not required for the patient's condition in order to make money. There are as many forms as there are physicians.

Direct cash kickback is probably where it started. If we're dealing with Medicare or Medicaid, anywhere there's direct reimbursement from the government or from private insurance companies, what the physician would want is some monies back after the laboratory collects the money from the insurer. I send you five hundred bucks worth of work, I get reimbursed. Two hundred fifty dollars for that travels back to me, the physician's office.

That's the way it was done at first, but then schemes developed. They developed the rotating-stocks schemes where they based the reimbursements or "dividends" back to the physician on the volume of lab tests that he sent in each day, or month, or what have you, whatever their accounting was. There was incentive to order more tests.

But then they had other things too. They had the free vacations in Hawaii, or use of cabins in Mammoth for skiing, or incentive trips to Europe. I've heard of things like paying for the doctor's office rent. Even paying for the kid's college—whatever you could think of, whatever way that comes to mind.

Some of this stuff gets too easy to discover now. If you pay the guy's rent, they're going to know who paid for it, there's a paper trail there. If you just give him cash, he'll pay his own rent and it ends there. Then there's other things like free tickets to basketball, football, any major sporting event, or season tickets to the opera.

When is it just an innocent gift, shall we say not related to excessively abusing the patient, and when is it definitely abuse in terms of raising more revenue? That's a big gray area. I don't see anything wrong in an occasional gift. I guess it's the magnitude of the reimbursement. But the stock games and picking up tabs, picking up car payments, picking up house payments, picking up school payments, picking up whatever. That's income. And basing it on the amount of business the physician provides, that determines whether it's a kickback.

What is the physician's role in laboratory fraud? Some physicians accept kickbacks from suppliers. This has been the case for as long as I can remember. It doesn't always have to be money. For instance, sex can be a payoff. In the big cities, hookers are offered as a bonus for referrals. The marketing man might take the doctor out on the town. A good looking gal might accompany them, and the doc might never suspect that she's from an escort service. He might never realize that it wasn't his line that got her into bed, but the telephone line to the answering service.

A nother technique to influence lab referral is sample supplies. The marketing rep will subtly ingratiate himself by providing office supplies. Another one is giving used equipment or selling it at a great discount. Of course the doctor doesn't know that the equipment is probably brand new. Free centrifuges are the favorite equipment to give away.

W hen you offer doctors automated chemistries at discounted prices, while billing insurance companies and patients at inflated prices, the doc's personal judgment is distorted. The whole question of medical necessity is compromised. The financial impact on the doctor is minimal, but everyone pays through the nose because these costs are passed on to the taxpayer.

S ome labs offer two free tests if the doctor orders a multiple test computerized analysis. The doctor is sent the results and bills the patient for all the tests including those at no charge to the doctor. Medicare and Medicaid patients—the same thing— billed for all the tests including the free ones.

T he latest gimmick in our area is the "Bandito" lab. Illegals from south of the border work in unlicensed clinical labs equipped with obsolete automated equipment that's still effective. Lab work is solicited from doctors with indigent non-English speaking patients. The doctor is charged a lesser amount than he can bill the insurers. He has a shell lab, which is a fake lab, set up in his own office to cover his tracks. The doctor than charges the full price based on manual testing, not automated.

W hen you go to a doctor's office, they'll draw the specimen and then they send it out to an independent laboratory. Two months later you may get a bill from this laboratory, but you're charged at the doctor's office also for drawing the blood and sending it out.

My husband went to a cardiologist and he had blood drawn. The doctor charged $80 for the blood to be drawn and wrote on the little slip all the tests that were to be done. Then we got another charge from the lab, and it was less. It was $47.

He got the two bills together and called the doctor's office and said, "I think you've double charged." They got really antsy. They called four times and apologized and said the bookkeeper made a mistake. The only reason he got any action is because he squeaked. Patients need to go over their bills with a fine-tooth comb.

7

QUALITY OF CARE

The threat from the business side of medicine doesn't lie solely in fraud—the people we talked to seemed to agree that when medical decisions are based primarily on business considerations, quality of care suffers greatly. Along those lines, we heard a great deal of worried speculation about the future of health care because of the pre-reform scramble to control costs. Yet it greatly encouraged us to see that although they were faced with uncertainty, the primary concern of those we spoke with was how to provide the personal attention and care required to meet the needs of their patients.

Quality of care issues encompass the whole range of medical practices and medical ethics, from how clean the floor of the operating room is to what kinds of sophisticated procedures are offered to extend life. Indeed, nowhere do all these issues come together more pointedly than at the end of life, and many of the comments in this chapter deal with that aspect of medicine, where quality of care can be equivalent to quality of life.

Nursing was as different in the old days as medicine was. It was individual care. Camaraderie for one thing. You cared about your staff and you cared about your patients. True, it was more limited in what you could do, but you had hands-on care of the patient. You can't tell me that a touch to someone who's ill from someone who cares doesn't make a difference. It makes all the difference in the world. And that one-to-one has gone.

And the problem is paperwork. Eighty-five percent of a nurse's time is spent on paperwork for government agencies. You're dying from the damn paperwork and where does the paperwork go? Not to the patient down the hall who needs you. I want to know, how much paperwork cures people?

But if you don't do the paperwork, you don't get the money. And money makes the hospital go around.

The one thing that we all noticed when Mr. Clinton gave his big speech was when he referred to the paperwork being done and the amount of time it took, he gave the impression that it was all insurance forms. Wrong. That's just a very small part of all the paperwork that we have to go through, and it's increasing daily.

In radiology we have nothing to do with insurance forms, and yet we're more busy taking the temperature on the refrigerators, we're being forced to do more paperwork to satisfy the JCAHO [Joint Commission on Accreditation of Healthcare Organizations]. And it almost seems like those people are inventing more paperwork and more projects for us to do to justify their position.

The paperwork in radiology alone has increased fifty to seventy-five percent in the last year over what it was the year before, which in turn was an increase over the year before. It's just been constantly escalating. If we get more government involvement, we're talking about even more paperwork—they go hand in hand. Already we're finding that our paperwork is interfering with our patient care. Who has time for a patient if you've got a report that's due?

I think it's quite ironic that we have all these government agencies requiring extensive reporting and documentation to ensure quality of care for the patient, and yet it's the very paperwork that those agencies have created that is reducing the quality of

care. Which one offers a higher standard of care, a nurse who's
with the patient at their bedside, who has the time to listen to the
patient, or the nurse who's sitting at the nursing station filling out
reports for some government agency?

When my husband was in the hospital, they had the unit
drugs right in the room. They're not supposed to make as
many mistakes, I guess. They have a lock, and they have to unlock
everything before they give you this medicine.

The first thing I noticed was that the nurses' aide brought in
the pills and set them down on the table and said, "Don't forget
to take your pills." A nurses' aide doesn't have the authority to
dispense meds, or the training either. I told my husband not to
take them. He was on Coumadin and I wanted to know if it was
the right dosage, so I hunted for an RN, and hunted, and hunted.
On that floor in the evening, I had a hard time finding one. When
I finally did, I said to her, "I'm concerned about my husband's
Coumadin/Sodium. A nurses' aide brought it in and just set it
down." The nurse said, "Oh, that's the right dose, I already
checked it." She didn't even come in the room. She didn't look
to see what it was. She didn't have time to talk with me. I guess
she was too busy doing paperwork.

The second error was, in my husband's room underneath the
sink was a washbasin. I was going to get it so my husband could
wash his hands. I looked down and here were more pills. There
was a couple Percadans and a vitamin and a couple others. All
those were in the wash basin. Tell me, why were those there?
When the nurses' aide came along, I said to her, "I found these
in the wash basin." She said, "Oh, thanks," and stuck them in
her pocket. She never even looked at them to see what they were.
She was probably embarrassed about it, and she wasn't going to
say anything about it. I bet no one was going to get an incident
report on it.

On top of all this, my husband was a little incontinent because
of all his medication, so they put a diaper on him. They called it
a diaper, which was quite humiliating for him. When I came in
one evening, I asked him if he had gotten up to go to the bath-

room, and he said, "No. They say I'm too slow. They told me not to bother."

Nobody has the time to take care of patients anymore. They had one RN on that whole floor. She should have been dispensing the meds. And besides that, they didn't even have the staff to help the patients get up to the bathroom. That's the kind of care you get in hospitals these days.

I was in the hospital a month ago and they wanted to give me medication through an IV, but they had already taken it out. I told them to just have it ordered by mouth, which I knew they could do. They wanted to keep me another day, but they couldn't get the IV back in so they had to send me home. Because of insurance requirements, I had to have an IV in or they wouldn't pay for another night. I wasn't feeling well enough to go home. I'm a nurse; I know when I need to stay another day.

The doctor no longer determines how long you'll stay in the hospital. It's Utilization Review. The doctor may want you there to keep an eye on you because he's suspecting a subdural hemorrhage, but that's tough, you go home. And then come back if you need to.

The man who lives next door to me builds the only ambulances on the West Coast. He makes money. He said that his business has picked up primarily in the last few years because all these patients are sent home so fast, they wind up being transported right back. Back and forth. It's created a need for more ambulances.

Hospital stays are really limited. You have to be in and out. We call it, "Quicker but sicker." Then in many cases, they come right back in through the emergency room within a matter of days, even hours.

When they bring you back into the hospital you have to go through the admissions process all over again. How many pieces of paper is that? Then you've got to make copies for this and copies for this and copies for that. And this goes here and that goes there. It ends up taking an hour and a half to admit somebody.

Why has it gotten this far? Why hasn't somebody been smart enough to stop it? You get too many agencies involved with too much money behind them. It's top heavy with government involvement.

I don't see how we can survive if increasing paperwork continues. The amount of nursing care given to paper is a horrendous amount.

I happen to be a computer buff, and I think that the computer is such a big answer to care and the riddance of a lot of paperwork. I long for the time when a health record could be on a little microchip, where people could bring that in and it would have their history and we wouldn't need to record as much as we do. On the other hand, until we get the lawyers out of the middle of that pot, I don't know how you're going to be able to eliminate the paper trail as we see it today.

I did hear a real story the other day that I thought was a great one. An individual had just returned from China. A new hospital was being built and they were patterning it after "the American system." I thought, oh, dear, what will that mean? The person who was telling this story was a person who came from a medical records background. This individual had been to China to help establish the medical records department in the new hospital.

One day while she was over there working, she fell and cut her head, which required stitches. The hospital that she was working on was not yet open, so she went to a hospital just down the street, not very far from where she worked. There was no anesthesia, but the suturing was done and she survived.

She was appalled that there was no medical record made of what was done. She was thinking in terms of medical records, and she said, "You know, I was just appalled that they didn't keep any medical records, so I asked them what they did about it. And they said, 'We only record that which is absolutely essential, and we know what's happening to you, so we haven't recorded that.' "

She wanted to know how many people that four-hundred-fifty-bed hospital had working in medical records, and was told they had two. She said, "I couldn't believe it. Here in this new hospital, which is a three-hundred-and-fifty-bed hospital, they have fifty-one individuals already hired to work in the medical records department because they've got to keep better records."

My heart just sank. I thought, here we are trying to help people in China, and what we're doing is infecting them with our problem areas.

F rankly, over the many years that I've taught nursing, I have always felt that by and large students are not motivated by personal gain. Rather, they're really motivated to do something worthwhile in life to help somebody else along the trail. On the other hand, it doesn't take long until their motivations begin to change.

I don't see that changing until about the time they graduate from the baccalaureate program. Then you begin to see how they begin to feel overwhelmed, and that the care that they want to give is impossible in the present situation. They get discouraged, and we see many individuals who leave nursing because they feel they are buried in paperwork, or that they're taking care of machines more than they are taking care of people.

They're not afraid of the intensive care components. They see that as important, but they're also caught with the ethical concerns of the unnecessary extension of life for both the young and the old. They question whether too much surgery is being done. I see that as an ethically philosophical issue with nursing down through the years, but much more increased during the last few years as we have seen a rise in technology.

I would say that in the majority of cases we spend our dollars on the other end of the spectrum, where we could probably do much better service if we started earlier. Quality of care should include what you prevent as well as how you treat it once it's happened.

The values in this society are for youth and beauty. Because we are a high-tech society, you value productivity. If you are no longer able to produce, you are a second class citizen. Right now, with the health-care costs going so high so fast, you're going to have to ration it somehow. If your value is productivity, the rationing will probably take place in the elderly population first.

Frankly, I think that we already have this two tier system. If you've got the money and you can pay well, doctors will look after you well. If you don't have the money, you're going to have to wait in this long line. HMOs are great, but you can't choose your doctors and they do everything to keep your elective surgeries down, and things like that. Now if you have the money, you can go to a private doctor. You can get a lot of things. They say you can't buy health, but poor health accompanied by wealth is certainly very helpful.

One of the problems we see in this country is that we clump the elderly all into one group, as if all the elderly were the very oldest, the last aged segment of this elderly population. When the news media talk about this elderly group as being so sick and using up all the health-care money, they're actually talking about the very old.

The elderly age range is the largest of any of our age segmented population. It goes from sixty to one hundred and past. That's a forty-year span. You can't really group them together. They're very different. The first ten years after retirement, from sixty-five to seventy-five, they're very healthy yet and they're productive. They can do lots of things. They've got lots of money and time for volunteering. The next one may not be quite that heavy, but they're still not burdensome. It's the last one, eighty-five and over, that is indeed the problem—the sickest, the poorest, and everything.

This whole group we label "elderly" is not using up all that health-care money, necessarily. It's a smaller segment, primarily the last segment of eighty-five and older. They use up a huge amount of money because of the long-term care costs that coincide because this group here uses the most long-term care. If you go to the long-term care, which is the nursing homes, you'll find that the average age is about eighty.

The biggest concern that the elderly have, and this is from research, is prolonged illness where they become dependent. I think the goal of the elderly people, and not just the elderly people, but society and everybody, is to keep them as independent and functional as long as possible, and keep them in their own homes as long as possible. I think that's everyone's hope.

I think Hillary Rodham Clinton's ideas are focusing in that direction, to provide as many community resources as possible to aid the families that care for these older people, and to help even the elderly couple in this society to maintain their health in the community. In fact just yesterday, I was giving this lecture about community resources, a social worker wanted to put this elderly couple in a nursing home, but the elderly couple did not want to go to a nursing home. They fought to stay in their own place.

It's more cost effective to keep the elderly at home and independent. Do you know how much it costs for them to go in a nursing home? Average? Thirty thousand a year. That's about $2,500 a month. That's out-of-pocket expense. Medicare picks up no custodial care. No insurance will pay for custodial care except Medicaid, if you're eligible.

They say if you're single, in about thirteen weeks or so you've spent down to poverty level because it costs so much. When you spend down until you're in the poverty level, then Medicaid will kick in. Even for a couple, although it takes a little longer than that, you'll spend down to where you become eligible. It's very expensive. Who can afford that, really, unless some level of government pays for it?

Our current system doesn't promote recovery, it almost makes the individual dependent on the health-care system for the remainder of their life. Insurance payments sometimes foster that kind of thing. They'll pay for the emergency room, but they won't pay for certain kinds of doctor's office visits. Or, they may pay if you're in the hospital for certain things, but not when you're discharged from the hospital. They'll pay for medication if you have been discharged from the hospital for so many days, but they won't just pay it for you for as long as you need it. Medicare offers no preventive care. They don't give you a physical. They don't give glasses or hearing aids or things like that. So if you don't have good glasses and you fall and fracture your hip, they'll pay for that, but not preventive kind of things like glasses.

I guess one of the biggest complaints I have about the system is that it's just too focused on terminal care and not focused enough on preventive care. That's my personal philosophy, and that's my professional philosophy as a nurse practitioner. I used to do Intensive Care Unit nursing for a number of years and lost a lot of patients and thought to myself, "I'm at the wrong end of this river here. And it's becoming a waterfall. Let's start out at the other end here and see if I can't make some difference." That's why I switched from ICU nursing to being a nurse practitioner and primary care because I wanted to make an impact so that maybe they didn't end up in an ICU.

Our medicine has gotten so good, we save a lot of children who before would have died due to these birth defects. Medicine is so accomplished, we are able to save them and allow them to live a full chronological life. But what about the quality of that life? We've addressed one issue, medicine is a wonderful thing and we've done tremendous things from that point of view, but we've kind of fumbled the ball afterward. We've allowed the mediocrity of just maintenance of a person who has a disability who survives birth and whatever other physical defect there is. We have allowed ourselves to become complacent and say that this is the quality of their life, and we feel that this is the best for them.

During Ronald Reagan's administration as governor here in California, he realized that a lot of money went into feeding and caring for people with disabilities, so he said, "We have to

take one segment of this group, and we have to say we can't serve
you anymore." And so, essentially the mentally ill people were
picked to lose services. And as a result, a lot of hospitals were
closed to these people and we weren't ready as a society to accept
them into the mainstream. They're the homeless. They're the
people who live under bridges. They're the people who just can't
normalize. They don't know where to get help. They feel ostra-
cized, and they really have been. They have been because we
don't know them. The doors of the hospital were opened and they
were requested to move on out.

But that's a travesty that we're haunted by now, right now.
There are very few services, and the services that are available are
totally and completely inadequate. Again, we're still going by the
same old mindset. We can't afford to provide the kind of service
that we've done before. But we don't need to. We don't need to
warehouse these people, because they've survived on the street
for many, many years. They've got a lot of skill that we don't
know about.

So many fantastic things have happened which have allowed
for the survival of a person, whereas before they would have
succumbed to the disease or the trauma. In that sense, we now
have the ability through the technology to assist a person to survive. On the other hand, what that has led to is just the maintenance of that person's life.

I applaud the efforts. I marvel at all the technology. I think it's
wonderful. But it can't stop at that point. I think it has to go on
into another realm and that is the care and nurturing of the individual after that.

Because of the number of patients that you're going to add,
and the inability of the system to handle that, they're going
to lower their standards. They want to lower the standards already. They want to do away with licensure for medical technologists.

In our hospital, the number of RNs per patient has gone down
strikingly. They've increased the number of nurses' aides and Li-

censed Practical Nurses. They feel that they don't need that highly trained person. A lot of times on some of our non-acute wards, there will just be one RN and the rest will just be aides and LPNs.

Now they can justify that up one side and down another, but the bottom line is that the quality of care is going to be affected. That's exactly what's going to happen. It's happening now.

There is nothing that you can do. If you're in a position of management in ancillary services, you do the best with what administration allows you to have. You try to find the appropriate places to substitute a licensed, college-trained person with somebody who's not. We try to be judicious in picking those people; that's the best you can do as a manager.

For the past fifteen years, I've worked in the blood bank in the laboratory. Right now, I'm the blood bank supervisor at a hospital. I've seen a lot in fifteen years.

It's become a lot harder. It's a completely different mentality. The people who are going into the field now are a completely different type of person. The people who have stayed have definitely broadened—this kind of sounds like a contradiction in terms—but broadened their specialties. In other words, they used to have one thing that they did very well. Now what we're looking at is people who have to be very good at a lot of different things. People are stretched thinner, work harder. This is hospital staffing. It's the future trend in health care—stretched thinner, worked harder.

People are leaving the health-care field left and right. There are not going to be any nurses. There are going to be fewer techs. The employee mix of a hospital now is going to foreign-trained. The number of people where English is the primary language is disappearing. I know some labs where you can walk in and no one speaks English.

The reason is simple. The trend in health care now is to hire people without benefits. This is the truth—I don't want it to appear that I'm a racist. It has nothing to do with that. It has to do with willingness of people to work for less. On the surface, it may not look like that, because they're earning a pretty good salary, but the big trend now is to hire a whole bunch of permanent part-time people without benefits.

There are a number of people out there in the health-care field that will work two or three jobs. That's the reality. They're willing to work two or three jobs and send half of their money home to another country. Those are the type of people that are flooding the market now. I don't think we've hired anyone full-time in ages. The number of those people who work a single job is dwindling fast.

These people don't have the same dedication to their primary job because they really don't have a primary job. You're going to have less quality. You're going to have people that are poorly trained with less experience. What we're going to create, and you can just see it, is a situation where the standard of care is going to end up much lower than where it has been.

You know, when I first started out in this business four years ago, I had an entirely different opinion of doctors. I thought, whatever a doctor told you, that must be the way it is. He gave you a diagnosis, and if that's the way he saw it, then he must be right. The doctor was always right and he always practiced with the highest integrity and care. Then I started going in the back rooms of some of the doctors' offices and seeing how they do business. For instance, when they autoclave their instruments, some of them weren't even soaking them and putting them in pouches. I was thinking, these guys are operating with these kinds of tools? Vaginal speculums—they're not autoclaving them. They're just rinsing them off and using them again. And these are supposed to be some of the finest doctors around. I'm seeing this and saying to myself, I wouldn't go into this doctor's office and allow them to do any procedures on me. There's no way.

I would say seventy percent of the doctors I work with, I have a great deal of respect for. Those are the ones that I think are giving good care and are really in it, not just for the monetary

reasons, but because they have a heart for people and they're trying to help. I think those seventy percent are excellent. Then there
are about thirty percent that I don't even think should be physicians. It's frightening.

When health-care reform comes to fruition and we're all in
managed care situations, I can really see different levels and qualities of care being practiced under the guise of a very controlled
and monitored system. We're not all going to be treated equally,
that's for sure. Some of us are going to be going to that thirty
percent of the doctors, the ones that, for example, hire unqualified medical assistants to give injections. It's very easy for them to
go to the medical cabinet and take an injectable drug, and they
think they've got the right one. I think a lot of mistakes are going
to happen as that thirty percent is trying to make as much money
as possible in a more efficient system.

I think the situation with physicians is going to be, you're going
to have the good ones retire or get out. Or you're going to have
some that will overwork and their quality is going to go down.
Then you also have the issue of the foreign-trained, the poor com-
municators, the poor quality physician.

The push to do away with specialties and going to general
practice type people is going to affect health care, too. You're going to have physicians forced to make medical decisions that they
probably wouldn't have made in the past. They would have referred them on to a specialist. Sometimes that's not good, but
sometimes it's darn right. It's another block that's going to go on
that side of the scale of poor quality health care and it's going to
be extremely frustrating.

I use this analogy with people who work for me at an entry level
in the laboratory, to explain to them consequences of their actions in health care. It's not like working for McDonald's where
if you don't get a hamburger right you throw it out—you're talking about people's lives.

And damn it, I'm of a real strong belief that you pay based on
acuity and consequence. That's why when I see them wanting to

cut costs and put less qualified people in positions of authority and control costs from a labor standpoint, I am dead set against it. This applies from the lab assistant with a high school education, all the way to the medical director. Their actions have greater consequences than someone who's a general contractor. Or someone who writes books for a living. You know if you don't get your first version right, you can go back and change it. If you don't spell words right, you've got spell check. In health care, a lot of times there isn't that luxury.

To get those high quality people, you have to pay money. So it becomes a vicious circle again. The new type of people that are coming into health care now are those that are willing to work for less money. They're not as qualified. They're not as dedicated.

O ne time when I was on call, I got called in the middle of the night. It was about two a.m. or so. When I came in, the entire parking lot was filled with street gangs. I went and shot the x-ray of the patient. This guy was just beaten to a pulp. He was bleeding out of every orifice he could possible bleed out of. He may even have had stabbing wounds, but the only thing that the ER doctor wanted was a chest x-ray and a skull x-ray.

I did the chest x-ray, then an anterior-posterior and a lateral—a front view and a side view of the skull. I noticed a skull fracture. You could see this nice little line going down. I took it back over to the ER doc, he looks at the films and says, "I'm letting this guy go. He doesn't have a pneumothorax. We've got to get rid of all these idiot people out here. There's nothing wrong with his skull. He's out of here. I'm getting all of these people out of here." He was worried about all these people rioting if they were told there was something seriously wrong. Maybe they would have torn the hospital apart, who knows.

I'm sitting there thinking to myself, should I say anything? should I not say anything? I go over and say, "Can I talk to you for a second?" He said, "No, I'm very busy." I said, "No, I have to talk to you for a second." I pulled him over here and showed him this little mark on the film and said, "Look, I'm not positive, but I've seen enough of these things. I think you need to keep this guy here, and I think that you need to send him over to (another hospital)." We didn't have a CT scanner at our hospital at the time, and he needed to go somewhere where they could take care of him.

They ended up calling the radiologist out that night to get a backup reading. Sure enough, he had a skull fracture and they transferred him. The guy was in ICU for three or four days. If they would have discharged him from the ER, he would have probably died.

It was just a lucky thing on my part, but at least I got him to call. With the ER guys, you really have to keep an eye out. They get tired and they get stressed out because they're managing the whole territory, plus seeing all these patients. Plus, they're trying to be eight different types of doctors. They need to be an orthopedic guy, they need to be a chest guy, they need to be a radiologist, they need to be a surgeon, they need to be a cardiologist, they need to be everything, and they lose sight of things sometimes. Good techs and good nurses really keep the ER guys out of trouble. Particularly when you go to the busy ERs.

M uch of how nursing is practiced, like in mega medical centers, is highly technical. It's very machine focused and I have a fear that our wages will price us out. If the dollar is going to be the major criterion, we're out. In our society, the medical profession still has the right to train anybody and be supervised by them. They tried it a few years ago with a registered technologist. They were going to train these people in two years to be able to monitor these machines and to do what they told them to do.

Nursing still has a role to do what the doctor orders, but we also have an independent role—diagnosing the human response. We focus on the human condition and then make a plan of care around alleviating that human condition. A machine and a technologist can't do that.

A t this point in time, we have so many people running frightened. We have the patients running frightened because they don't know if their health care is going to be lessened tomorrow.

We have hospital administrators that are frightened because hospitals have become more or less, corporations, not care givers. We're running on a budget line, we're not running on a patient care line anymore. Maybe what we need to do in the United States is go through a drastic change and get health care back to where we don't have to run along a budget line in place of the patient care line.

I can speak to the fact that many of our acute cases that had been in the hospital and then sent home for care, many of those where the spouse or whoever was able to give the care needed, cut the costs tremendously, and the patient moved along very well on the wellness standpoint. That needs to be paid for, and it's much cheaper than to keep the patient in the hospital. There's got to be flexibility in the system, and I don't know how we're going to do that.

One of the issues that medicine is looking at these days is the concept of futile care. No matter what we do, it's not going to help improve the quality of life. If it's not going to help improve the medical condition, at what point do we stop medical care? I think the greatest percentage of health-care dollars are spent in the last 350 days of a patient's life. So, is what we're doing futile? At what point do we stop?

One doctor explained futile care to me, and I really found it very enlightening. If you were sick and you needed to be on an antibiotic, and he gave you a particular antibiotic—Antibiotic A—and you weren't responding to it, the doctor has the right to stop that antibiotic and try something else. Or maybe not try anything else. The doctor makes that decision. It would be futile to continue with Antibiotic A if it wasn't doing any good.

That's how we should look at medicine. The doctor at this time has not been given the authority or decision making to deem medicine futile. The family makes that decision. In the scenario I just used, does that patient still decide that he wants Antibiotic A even though it's doing no good? Does the patient have the right to make that decision?

We need to educate the public as to when medicine is no longer effective, and at what point do you allow a patient to have death with dignity. I've found very often, at least in the intensive care unit, so much of what we see has to do with allowing patients to die with dignity. If a patient is in an intensive care unit, they have tubes hooked up to every opening of their body. Their body is exposed to the world. It's not very dignified. And if we then have to initiate CPR, we are physically beating up their body. It's not a pretty picture.

Some patients will say they want that anyway, and yet we forget that death is a part of life. It's a continuum. It starts at birth, in the middle is adolescence and young adult, then adult, middle-aged, and aged. Then comes death. It's part of the timeline and part of the spectrum and we lose sight that it's part of the process. After all this is going to come death. We have difficulty accepting that.

I think that for many people, death is terrifying. Yet we as a culture and a society, and even the microcosm of the medical team, can make death a very comfortable process. It doesn't have to be scary. It doesn't have to be ugly, and it doesn't have to be traumatic. It can be actually very pleasant, if you will. I'm not proposing euthanasia. I'm talking in terms of futile care.

"Pleasant" may sound like such a horrible term to say, but I personally witnessed a family member experience a very pleasant, comforting death. It wasn't ugly. I left feeling satisfied and comfortable that he was now comfortable. I think we sometimes lose sight of that, and we strive so hard to continue life that that struggle is very ugly for the patient.

D octors have the highest death anxiety of any professional group. Terminal patients make doctors anxious and force the attitude of, do everything possible to extend life, regardless of quality.

A nurse taught me there is nothing wrong with dying. She knew when it was time for the patient to go. She would mention the patient by name and ask me, "Should I bathe the patient and turn him on his side?" There was no euthanasia. She made the patient comfortable, and then waited for the end.

I'm not for euthanasia. I'm not for early death because life is difficult. But, I think there are many times when a life is extended beyond that which it should be, and to the detriment to both the patient and the caretakers.

I don't think I ever saw anybody who was pulled that shouldn't have been pulled. It was the most humane thing to do. I don't think I ever saw one that was inhumane. Everyone finally comes to an agreement that, yes, we need to let this person die because that's inevitable right now. Medicine has done all it can.

Some doctors do too much for the terminally ill. It's not because they are greedy, but because they are afraid of failure. Their entire education stressed technical skills. The human skills of accepting death as an inevitability are lost.

Doctors have a mixed bag of feelings around genuinely sick elderly patients. They don't want to accept defeat of their medical skills and they feel comfortable dealing with really sick patients. Their natural fear of death makes the doctor take the extra step if only to delay the inevitable. Why do you think that most health-care dollars are spent during the last years of life? Why do you think that most doctors are unalterably opposed to rationing care and permitting the elderly and the disabled to die?

There has to be a decision on the part of the medical team that asks, "Do you think this person's life will be bettered?" I know many individuals who I have seen have surgery, who everybody on the medical team would have said the chance of this person getting better is nil. It might extend their life more comfortably for a few months, but is that worth the risk or cost? We must be made to show indications that it is.

We treat our animals better than we treat human beings. If I am diagnosed with lung cancer and it's metastasized to my brain and my bones and all through my body, why would I want to have some guy say, "We're going to give you six weeks of chemotherapy followed up by radiation therapy, and we're going to open up your skull and take the tumor out." In the final analysis, once that disease has metastasized, you're done. You might as well get yourself in order and have the doctor give you medication for pain, and do the best you can to die with some dignity. Not go into some hospital and have them run up thousands, hundreds of thousands of dollars, in treatment for something that's going to have the same net result, which is, you're going to die.

I see that, more and more, our patients and our families are moving in the direction of no heroic measures, no CPR, no ventilator support. Wanting death to be as comfortable and painless as possible. We as a hospital really strive for comfort and dignity. That's very important to us. By the same token, if there's that opportunity for life and living, if we see there's an opportunity for some quality of life and a chance to really help a person move in that direction, we want to offer them that opportunity as well.

Sometimes we're maintaining life support on people who really need to have the opportunity to die. I've been in ethics committee meetings, and there were times when you had to call a family in, with one member really not wanting to let this family member go, and you had to convince them this person needed to die. Their whole body functions were gone and you're doing all sorts of things to prolong a life that's essentially already ended. A lot of us nurses say we're going to tattoo something across our chest—"Don't ever put me on a ventilator."

A lot of us also talk about having another nurse, an intensive care nurse, be our living will with our family. I would never want my mom being in charge of my medical treatment. She would want to prolong my life, even if my life was not intended to continue.

I t seems to me so many people are unwilling to die. And yet we come into this life knowing we're going to end that way. We live in such a quick-fix society that wants everything taken care of for us. Our society is so used to the easy answer for everything. I want everything now. I want to be happy now. Do for me, and do it now.

P eople don't understand. They think you're there to simply make life go further. You're going to create this miracle, and this person's going to pull out and they're going to live happily ever after.

I remember seeing a lady who came in with severe cirrhosis and was on a respirator. She was in a coma. We were telling the family that this lady was probably going to die. She had been an alcoholic for years. Well, this lady pulled out of it. Although she came out of this episode, it didn't mean she wouldn't go into another one as soon as she had another drink. At that point, I don't think medicine enhanced her life. Unless the patient made some drastic changes, all we did was prolong her suffering by keeping her alive.

Y ou can make the lungs breathe. You can keep a brain-dead person alive for some time. You can have brain stem function, which is a complete vegetative state with no conscious cognitive actions at all, but the brain stem continues to send impulses to the heart to keep it going. Yes, you can keep a person going a long time in that state. If there weren't respirators around, this person would have died the natural course. But there is a point when all your efforts can do nothing to keep the heart and lungs going.

It's a real hard ethical question. Do you put someone on life-support in the hope that something happens to reverse it? If you answer yes, then you have to ask yourself, how long?

8

PRIMARY CARE IS A PRIMARY CONCERN

To most people we spoke with, quality of care hinged upon the quality of the personal relationship between the health-care provider and the patient. Unless that relationship is founded and nurtured, the patient could receive the finest testing and the most advanced therapy, the most accurate paperwork and documentation, but would still rate quality of care as poor. Those we interviewed agreed that the relationship would benefit from a renewed emphasis on primary care, from changing the focus from end-of-life care to preventive medicine, and recently there has been a shift of resources and personnel from specialized medicine. But the impetus has been financial, the focus has not been on quality of care, so it is difficult to tell what the benefits will be.

R emember when you had a GP and he took care of everything? You went to him for everything. One check and that was it.

Y ou can ask some patients, "Who's your doctor?" And they'll answer, "Well, which part of the body do you want? I've got a head doctor, I've got a chest doctor, I've got a knee doctor, and I've got a back doctor."

A similar thing happens in the women's health field. You've probably seen it advertised a lot—the Breast Center. So now women are just going to take their breasts somewhere? Right? I mean let's just ship one piece of our body off here and another piece over there. We have PMS centers and breast centers and menopause centers, but we don't have a total body center. Holistic health comes out of the health food store now.

It's definitely a complicated issue. How do you draw the line on who needs a test and who doesn't need it? It's become strictly a money issue. I'm thirty-seven years old, an ex-smoker. I think it's in my best interest to know what my body is doing. If nothing else, I'd like a baseline test or two to compare with down the road if I ever do develop a problem. If I already have the beginning of a problem, then I've probably got a better chance for early treatment before it ends up being a full-blown surgery or whatever.

I'm for preventive medicine where people know where they're going, know what their body's doing, letting the physicians kind of open you up, read the book and see what's inside there before bringing them in on the last chapter. We need to monitor things on more of a long-term basis.

I know Hillary's ideas are bent toward an emphasis on the generalist practice of medicine with a de-emphasis on the subspecialist. I happen to be a subspecialist, and I function in a setting in which there is quite an emphasis on the subspecialist practice of medicine. Medicine is so broad, that it is difficult for someone to function with excellence over this broad spectrum. I'm really far more economical in the practice of medicine in dealing with a very narrow spectrum, mine being hematology.

I had a very complex patient a few weeks ago with cardiac disease and pleural effusions built up on the top of Hodgkin's Disease. I took care of the Hodgkin's Disease. A cardiologist took care of the pericardial effusion, and a pulmonary subspecialist took care of the pleural effusions. We managed the patient together beautifully. I honestly don't know how a generalist could possibly manage a patient like that. In my particular medical group, in as much as there is not a particular emphasis on the general practice of medicine, I think we can function with more excellence in this fashion.

What happens in our whole fragmented care, people end up not being seen by the same person or being seen by so many different specialists that it ends up costing us more money, because nobody's putting that all together for them. Nobody's telling them, "Dr. So-and-so gave you this medicine, and then Dr. So-and-so gave you this medicine, which is exactly the same medicine, so you're double dosing. It may have a different name, but it's exactly the same medicine." Nobody's putting that all together and it ends up costing, costing in terms of health and costing in terms of money.

There's a difference between the kind of doctor who works the ER and one who has a private practice. I think they're more oriented to the here and now. They don't need to know this big, lifelong history. It's not important to them what's always been going on. Generally it's, you come in now, I see you now, and that's it. I'm done. My job has been fulfilled. An assembly line type thing. I don't think they have attitudes toward that, but I just think that's what they're geared for.

So they're not focused towards the whole long-term approach to a patient. If a patient comes in with one thing, they're going to treat that one thing. Every once in a while a patient will bring up, "By the way, this and this . . . " but the ER doctor says, "But that's not why you're here today. You're here for this, and this is what we're treating." I don't think that's either good or bad, but that's the rules.

A primary care physician has a more holistic approach to a patient, a more long-term relationship. We try to encourage all these people, who come in without doctors, to get doctors. It's silly for someone to come in chronically with a problem and only see an emergency room physician. They're not likely to see the same physician twice. They work all different hours, and their schedules are very erratic. You're not going to see the same doctor on a regular basis. Don't expect it.

We treat the parts and not the sum of the whole. I think it also expands beyond medicine to our culture. We no longer have families. We no longer have what we know as the unit family. Between divorce, people not even getting married, people so mobile and moving around. Families now, if there is a husband and a wife, both have to work. I think our concept of family has changed. As that has changed, the family doctor has changed. We no longer have the family practitioner. My own doctor is a specialist in family medicine, and I think it's wonderful. But we have fewer and fewer family practitioners because there's fewer and fewer families.

I am a nurse. However I've been in educational administration through a lot of my life also, because I'm very interested in educating the future health-care deliverers. With all of that, obviously I'm interested in quality health care.

As I look back on it, one of the things that I see as a strength from the past, which I see us recycling to, is the emphasis on the family's role in maintaining quality health. The emphasis on the parental role in terms of teaching children to care for themselves. Way back in the days when my mother was a public health nurse, I can remember her having family groups together, teaching mothers on parenting. At that time, she was paid through Metropolitan Life insurance. That was the old way that nursing in the community was cared for. Why? Because they recognized that it paid to pay for preventive health care.

And yet we went away from that. It is very sad when I see home health care, for example, has not been reimbursable by many, many health-care plans. If it were, we could do more preventive care. We could cut costs of delivery of health care to patients after acute illnesses if reimbursement were available to families who help themselves.

We have a lot further to go for the future in terms of getting families and individuals to care for themselves. There are many families that do not have role modeling at all from individuals who really know what health-care provision is, explaining that health care begins before the baby is born and health care involves all the family members.

Today there are individuals, up through the high school level, who have become so dependent on emergency care which is care for those who are bleeding, care for those who are in acute settings, care for those where if the child is sick enough, we'll do something about it, otherwise go home. There are many who have been brought up in that mode, who are not ready for taking responsibility for themselves. I think that's one of the things that needs to be nurtured.

I don't think that a lot of our system of doctor-driven health care helps us to examine what could be done by people themselves. I believe that one of the things that's helping that is nursing, nursing as a profession. Nurses have been one of the big proponents of this over the years, but their voices have not been heard. The rise today of more nurse practitioners will assist in helping, from pregnant women to their children to the whole family constellation in caring for themselves. There are others on the health team involved, but I've really seen nurses as the primary instigators and coordinators of health care in the home.

I can remember a few years ago dealing with a client who had a laryngectomy who just wasn't getting well. I finally went to the doctor who was caring for this man and said, "This patient is not far from where I'm seeing some other patients. How about if I went into the home and see what's going on in that home." Well hesitantly, he finally agreed, as though, go visit if you like, be it a charitable visit.

What a difference making that home visit. I found that the man had just recently lost his wife, he had no support system at home. He didn't know what laryngectomy care really meant. I was able to get this patient to see more laryngectomy patients so he could see some hope. We got that thing turned around. It wasn't any magic that I did, but it was insight from seeing the home situation.

That doctor said, "Boy, I can't believe what you did." Well, it wasn't anything that you as an individual can do, it's your overview of the whole.

H olistic medicine treats the whole body, not only the physical body, but the emotional body and the spiritual body. We don't do that in medicine. We have looked so much at traditional medicine, but what about the nontraditional? I believe one of the major insurance companies has now finally approved the nontraditional approach to cardiac disease, coronary artery disease; nonsurgical, nontraditional intervention including health, diet, exercise, spiritual, holistic intervention. It's a whole program and it takes about fifteen weeks. They have found success with it. You can do nonsurgical intervention and have the same success rate as surgical intervention. But I think it's so threatening because of the dollar.

I 'm working in the area of rehabilitation. My agency works with individuals who have either some traumatic brain injury or a developmental disability like mental retardation or cerebral palsy or epilepsy. Typically the other processes are such that this person will be institutionalized and stay there forever and ever and ever and never have an opportunity to try anything on their own. I worked in these hospital settings, small board and care centers. We were doing the same repetitive things over and over and over for years and charging the state an exorbitant amount of money to do this same thing. In addition to that, they were doing a behavior modification programming. For what? You're going to modify someone's behavior so they can live in an institution better the rest of their lives?

What we do is we abandon the whole notion that a person has to be given services in an institution or in a classroom setting or any other kind of segregated type of arrangement. We work to integrate the person into the community. We find out what they want for themselves in the long run, and we take this script and plug in the services that are necessary for them to be successful. We're proving time after time, people with some serious problems can learn to integrate into a community given a chance. The thinking has been that eventually this adult will become proficient at managing their own life, we don't need to be there anymore, and we'll fade in certain areas until they become totally independent. That's a tremendous cost savings, the person is now living a more normalized life.

As they become successful, it just snowballs to the point we don't have to pay anyone to provide specialized services or training or board and care or anything for this person. We're talking minimal interface—maybe even zero dollars expended—from thousands and thousands of dollars a month. This person takes control of their own life and the state gets out and saves a whole bunch of money.

The insurance companies have seen it working now for the last few years and they're saying, "Hey, we realize the benefit of this. Number one, this person is now going to be integrated into the community and not institutionalized. And number two, we're not going to have to pay the kind of service fees we've had in the past."

I think this is where my disappointment lies in the system as it is. Rather than care being a total heartfelt service delivery system, people have found ways to gain a lot of money from warehousing people. Billions of dollars are spent annually in our state in caring for people with disabilities. It's not a grandiose idea that we had, this community integration, but it's never been developed because you can't get rich doing it. A lot of people would shy away from this kind of service because until recently, you could make a very, very healthy living providing real basic services to another human being, but not looking at their life as a whole. They were just numbers and in many cases still are. They fill a bed. They fill a slot. They are income. You could negotiate a rate of reimbursement that was quite high and it was lucrative to keep that person there.

When you have such an avant-garde kind of program like we have, it draws the ire of a lot of people, especially the old guard who are established in their care giving. A lot of folks are skeptical. A lot of people are certainly afraid of what might happen. Because of all of these "what if's," we continue to shoot ourselves in the foot. We're not allowing an individual to grow as a human being and a person.

I t used to be that the general practitioner could do surgery, deliver babies, take care of the colds and everything. That's much less so now. However under the direction that a lot of people are advocating, maybe we'll go back to more of that. There's a feeling that there's much too much specialization now and not enough general practitioners. Perhaps if we train more general practitioners they will be doing more of the minor surgery and uncomplicated deliveries.

M y first job was in 1962 in the city of Los Angeles. I worked in the south-western section which was mainly black at that time as it is now. I was what we call a general public health nurse, assigned a district, a boundary area within the city. We were given all the health referrals that needed contact in the home for follow-up and continuity of care. We would see teens who had babies and try to see that their postpartum was uneventful and that they had the support that they needed. We tried to encourage them to stay in school. Then we would do teaching about how to care for the baby and parenting and that kind of thing.

In other families that we saw, there might be someone recovering from tuberculosis. There was supervision, that they were following the medical regime, that they understood about their limitations. We had referrals from the city's health department so that every month we saw mothers who were going to deliver a baby. We would review what to expect in the next month, and then we'd look for complications in pregnancies.

We got the reportable communicable diseases. Public health nursing went out there and did the teaching about what kind of follow-up was needed. If they were having trouble accessing care we helped them in that arena to get the care that they needed. Then we'd see the multi-problem families, the poor, the people who were powerless, the people that didn't use the medical or social resources that were there in the community, or that used them and abused them.

We would review our caseload periodically with our supervising nurse. That was the person that decided, depending on our judgment, whether they should continue to be followed or whether they should be closed to this public health nurse supervision aspect. I think we carried a caseload of anywhere from 180 to 230 families in this area. We also had assignments to do counseling.

Some families you saw intensively maybe once a week for a period of time. Other families you saw maybe every three months. Some, like typhoid carriers, we only saw once a year. You could set your priorities, depending on what the family priority was and manage it quite adequately.

There were other assignments like doing the counseling in a clinic, like the prenatal clinic or the TB clinic or child health clinic. We would see that mother after the child received the physical exam, after they got their immunizations, after they got the doctor's instructions. Then we would have the time to sit with them for a few minutes and make sure they understood what the doctor said to them and check that they had the supplies to do what the doctor said, before they went back home. So we would review what the procedure was. Some of those that we felt needed a little more follow-up, we would write out a referral that the nurse that had the district where they lived went out to see them in a week or whatever, to help them accomplish the health goals that were needed at the time.

That was the kind of public health nursing role that I entered into and it is much different today. Today, the traditional prevention programs—there are still things that are funded—but like tuberculosis is followed completely by nurses that are employed in that tuberculosis clinic. They meet with the client at the clinic site. They may do follow-up over the telephone, but it's the client who comes to the clinic for any kind of supervision at all. There just isn't that kind of monitoring out in the home site. Today, they'll get their information over the phone, not face-to-face, unless the patient comes to the clinic site. They do their teaching over the phone.

Only three percent of the health-care dollar goes to prevention. The money does not flow to health departments as it has in the past. It was cut in the early eighties. Plus that's when the medical establishment was beginning all these high-tech organ transplant kinds of stuff so they were grabbing all the money for these major high-tech things. So there isn't a lot of money coming to nursing to do public nursing anymore.

The whole cycle of poverty is such that it's real hard to maintain a good level of health and so they utilize services more often too. I think they utilize services more often because they're also looking for more than just fix my ear or throat. It's more like, "Help me fix my life." So you see them more and the appointments take longer. It becomes a financial nightmare when you're getting reimbursed so little.

If they go to the emergency room to use their Medicaid and it's not an emergency condition, they're told that this is not appropriate use of the emergency room. Then they're expected to go someplace else for care. How do they get there? They don't have a car that works. They don't have money for gas. So problems just escalate. They just get worse and worse. And get more costly.

The system doesn't make it easy for people that are poor. They wind up in the emergency room for everything, and that only helps to increase fragmentation. It's more costly in the long run because they don't feel like they belong anyplace. They never see the same person twice, problems don't get attended to in a timely way and they end up more costly.

The general public thinks we can fix more than we can because of all of our technology. As it's been said many and many a time, we spend more than any other country in health care and we still aren't a healthy people. The last time I heard, we're twenty-fifth on infant mortality in the world. That's shameful. And that upsets me a lot. We do all of this expensive end-care, and we don't even help moms and babies have a good start.

High-risk infants become a major problem in the community, not only in their infant and preschool years, but for the school system. A public health nurse can do much to help that mother parent a high-risk child who doesn't have a neurological system that's intact, that needs really special individualized care in order to prevent some delays and lags down the road.

There's lots of funds available when that child is in the neonatal intensive care nursery across the street. They may come out with these humongous bills that without state and federal money some families would never make it. But then they go home and they don't have the support to help parent these children. To help them have a somewhat normal life. Putting money into prenatal care would prevent some of that.

We had a health fair here the other day, and I did breast exams for the health fair. When I got here at eight o'clock, there was already five people waiting. There was always five or ten people waiting the whole morning. I finished at twelve-thirty and then somebody else did them the rest of the afternoon. The reason the majority of them were here was they didn't have insurance and they didn't have any money. They were here to get whatever kind of health services they could at a cost they could afford. Women were coming in who had not had any kind of health care in five or ten years, who are moving into that higher risk age group, thirty-five to sixty. That's who's really losing out in the system.

A lot of times those people are moms, and a lot of times they're single moms. They'll spend the money on their kid. This happens frequently. They'll bring the kid in with a cough, and the mom's sitting there obviously much sicker than the child, but she brought the child in for the care.

If you look at the costs of the preventive aspects of care, and we know that we get a healthy baby when the mother has enough food, when she takes her prenatal vitamins and gets adequate iron for that infant. The babies that come out weigh more, they have a better fighting chance at life when they are born.

It's very significant that we have better health when our social system is intact, when we have food for the people, when there's medical care when they need it, when the environment is safe, when sanitation is in order. Those social kinds of necessities are important for health, too, and for positive health outcome. Nursing is concerned with caring, and I think part of the caring is thinking about the total human condition, seeing and being concerned that people have what they need.

I n seeing the prenatal patient in the home, that affects her worth as a person, and so therefore it helps her feel better as a person if you develop a trusting kind of relationship. I think we have a decrease in the abuse, battering and neglect of the child because they have made a connection. We need to develop a long-term relationship with the patient, rather than episodic care where nobody knows them. That's a role that the public health nurse used to play.

N urses have less and less time to spend with the patients. And part of the reason for that is the way we've structured our payment system. Nurses got thrown in with the room rate. You pay several hundred dollars a day supposedly for the room, the linen, food, housekeeping, the heat, and the nurses. Maybe because it's a female dominated profession, but nurses have never organized themselves well for their own good as a profession.

Doctors did. Doctors have more legal authority and clout in this country than most of us realize. I don't know how many people understand that a doctor could pull anyone off the street into their office, tell them to wash their hands, and then let them suture people up, examine people—anything the doctor wants—they can legally do that. It's all under the physician's license.

A nurse on the other hand has very restricted practice capabilities by law. She has a license for everything she can do. Because there was a great need for nurses a number of years ago, the nurses complied. So they said, "We'll try to squeeze all of nursing into two years instead of three years." Now we've ended up in a situation where nurses really don't have very much clout.

A nurse practitioner is a registered nurse with advance preparation. I have my master's degree in nursing. Really we're primary care and we are mostly preventive health. A big portion of what I do is ill care, but within that format of ill care we always have a philosophy of preventive health and also of health education, teaching people how to get well, how to stay well, and how to take care of themselves. Also, a big part of my practice is women's health. I've been in practice in this area for twelve years. In essence, I've been here longer than any of the physicians. I have the most longevity here.

Why would someone come to a nurse practitioner? Nurse practitioners tend to spend more time talking with people and helping them understand what's going on with them, helping them understand the health-care system. We have more time. We take more time. We also see our role as not a cure role but as an enabling kind of role, helping people stay independent and make independent decisions.

Sometimes people aren't able to find that with a physician. They're not able to find that time. They're not able to find that equality often. It's more often a patronizing kind of system from physicians. And it's also cure oriented. There's a lot that we can't cure. If you're taught how to cure something, but then you come up against things that aren't curable, you end up getting a little frustrated when you can't just say, "Here, take this and you'll be fine." It takes a lot more discussion and time. A nurse practitioner takes the time for that.

There are more jobs for nurse practitioners than can be filled because there's just not that many physicians going into family practice anymore. There's a big need for people in primary care. The people that are going into family practice aren't going into family practice in small communities. They stay in large groups. They stay in urban settings. They don't go into small communities. There are lots of rural communities that don't have any physicians at all. The nurse practitioner is often recruited for that. It's also financially easier to maintain a nurse practitioner than a physician.

You hear that time and again that there just isn't that country doctor anymore, there isn't that family doctor. There are, but a lot of people in an urban setting aren't able to find them. Or if they do find them, those doctors are so busy with HMOs they end up having to see patients every seven minutes. Well, what can you do with a patient in seven minutes? You can hardly say, "Hello. How are you? How's the family?"

Nurse practitioners are real cost effective. Our education is far less expensive and our expectations of remuneration aren't as great. So we are cost effective in that way. There was just a major study that came out that showed the cost effectiveness of nurse practitioners. And actually, in the health-care reform bill, they've been talking a lot about utilizing nurse practitioners. It's good to hear.

Nurse practitioners started twenty-five years ago in Colorado at the University of Colorado. At that time, it was projected that there was going to be a shortage of primary care physicians. There was going to be a shortage of physicians, period. They couldn't educate them quickly enough. They had seen how core people had worked in the wards and that worked really well. It doesn't necessarily take all the high-tech knowledge that a physician gets in order to take care of a sore throat, an earache, bronchitis, pap smears, women's health, contraception, teaching people preventive health, health education. So that was where the concept sprung from. Over the years it's evolved that nurse practitioners are more cost effective. We're also more available to a community.

It's not that we have a shortage of physicians, we have a maldistribution of physicians. They're in urban settings and they're in specialties, and they're all in competition with each other trying to get the same patients.

There isn't any glamour in going into family practice. They're not remunerated, which is what our society bases respect on. It's how much do you get paid for what you do. They're not, so they're not respected in that way, and they're not talked about as a need. Since we moved away from the family physician and primary care, in many people's minds you don't go to primary care. If you need a physical, you go to an internist. We need to re-educate the public.

On the other hand, a lot of people, especially the elderly, say to me, "I need a family practice doctor. I need my own doctor that's going to help explain all of this to me and help me negotiate the health-care system," because that's really very difficult for people. Like the other day, I was talking to a patient. She had gone to see an orthopedist because she was worried that she had osteoporosis. It hadn't been diagnosed. She just was worried because she had a family history of it. So he took an x-ray and he told her, "Yes, you have some osteoporosis starting, take some calcium, and walk." But he didn't talk to her about other things that I ended up talking with her about.

She also has a thyroid problem. She was taking way too much thyroid which robs the bones of its density. He didn't know that. That's not his job to know that. He's an orthopedist. He didn't know that the reason she was probably developing so much osteoporosis was because she wasn't balanced with the thyroid. And he didn't tell her about estrogen because he's not a gynecologist. And he didn't tell her about exercises and weight bearing and posture, and how important all that is, not just to walk, but to improve everything. So she said to me, "How come he didn't tell me any of this?" And I said, "You should have gone to primary care. That's the role of primary care."

People don't know that unless they experience it, so they don't know what they're missing. Instead, they keep fragmenting themselves out.

With insurance now, we've become the gatekeeper, which really makes a lot of people angry. Primary care is the gatekeeper as to whether you're going to see a specialist. It makes a lot of patients angry who are used to, "Oh, I've got something here on my skin. I better call the dermatologist," or "Gosh, I'm worried about osteoporosis. I'll go see an orthopedist." Now see, if she had insurance that wouldn't allow that, then that really would have saved the system some money because we could have handled all of that in primary care.

T he family physician died out for a number of reasons, primarily financial. And people, our whole health-care system, became enamored with high tech. The newest and the latest. That's why drug companies will market it as the newest and the latest. People now expect the latest technology, the latest CAT-Scan, the latest MRI, whatever. Our whole measure of value in health care is "the newest," "the latest," "the best."

You can go to a high-profile clinic to get a total complete physical. You can get the same health care from your primary care provider at one-tenth the cost with a lot more education and a lot more understanding that goes with that, than if you are just an anonymous person going to a high-profile clinic. But people really think that that's "the best." You hear it advertised on the radio. "Come for your executive physical."

People think that if you're not going to a specialist, you're not getting the best care. But then sometimes they get frustrated going to specialists because they still aren't getting what they want. Many specialists are good about trying to talk in people language, but many of them don't feel that that's their role at all. They feel that their role is to diagnose what the patient came there for and let primary care explain it. But then, people don't come back to primary care and have it explained to them. The gatekeeping function is a benefit to people. I know that it's hard for them to change because they feel a lack of independence, but it really is to their benefit.

I hope people are beginning to realize that we've paid a price in not looking at the total person. The consumer is not getting what they need. They're not getting their questions answered. They're not getting the education that they should have.

The physicians' reaction to nurse practitioners really varies depending upon the geographic setting and whether the person is primary care or specialty. In a lot of instances we're an economic threat. There's also ego involved. If somebody chooses to see a nurse practitioner, the reaction can be, "But she's a nurse practitioner. Why would you choose to see a nurse practitioner when you can see a physician?"

The reason is, we're meeting whatever needs that particular physician wasn't meeting in that patient. It's really an individual kind of thing. Not all nurse practitioners meet everybody's needs, and not all physicians meet everybody's needs. Fortunately, there's a bit of all of us to go around. But in some areas we're seen as a definite economic threat.

More and more nurse practitioners are going into private practice, going into solo practice all across the nation. That's generating a lot of hostility especially in a setting where there's not enough patients to go around.

I think that there's also a core of physicians that think nurse practitioners really have a place in the health-care system. They're supportive of us and support our role and recognize that we offer something different than what they're offering. They see that all of us are needed in this system.

A lot of people are real familiar with nurse practitioners, especially within the big HMO systems. A lot of people say, "Oh yes, I had a nurse practitioner before. She was my health-care provider." There's people that choose to see me because I'm a nurse practitioner, because they've had positive experiences before with nurse practitioners. A lot of women come to me for women's health because of my reputation in the community which I've built over a long period of time. And there's a lot of women that come to me because I'm a woman. That's my main qualification for many women who choose me.

Doctors tend to focus on their specialty, though some doctors now are beginning to broaden their spectrum and go back to generalized medicine. That's going to be the trend. Various educational programs now are offering reductions in student loans if they go and work as country doctors in family medicine, treating the whole versus the part. That's a trend we're going to have to move toward in the future to be effective.

Ophthalmology is in a sense a secondary level of care. While it's important for people with eye problems to be checked by an ophthalmologist to rule out the possibility of eye disease

and to get the care they need, not all aspects of eye care have to
be performed by an ophthalmologist. Glasses are the best example. An optometrist often does a better—and more cost effective—
job of prescribing glasses simply because an ophthalmologist's
training does not concentrate on simple refractions. They don't
get an awful lot of that in residency, they're concentrating on eye
disease and eye surgery. In fact it's becoming more common for
an ophthalmologist to team up with an optometrist so they can
offer the best and most cost effective service in eye care.

I had many years of a bad back. Being an x-ray technician and
then in medical equipment sales, I knew a lot of chiropractors,
a lot of medical doctors, a lot of orthopedists. I knew the good
ones and the bad ones.

I would go to the chiropractor any time I would injure my back
and within two or three visits I was up and walking around again,
because he's dealing with muscles and tendons and bones. And
he's a damn good physiotherapist, and his hot pack is as good as
any medical doctor's hot pack. His diathermy is as good as any
medical doctor's diathermy. And he's got to work harder because
he can't give me any pain pills.

But there came a time when I came in and I told the chiropractor
what had happened. I had a real flare-up and I had numbness down
my leg. He said, "I don't think I'm going to help you this time.
You've got to go to an orthopedist. You need surgery. You've either
got a ruptured disk or some disk material that's torn off." It turns
out it was torn off and lodged against the sciatic nerve.

You see there's a chiropractor that knows his limitations and
he had treated me for ten years, but there came a point where
that treatment wasn't going to help. Now I might have gone to a
doctor, and if I'd gotten the wrong orthopedist I would have been
under the knife nine years earlier. Would it really have been necessary then? No doubt I needed it when I did have it done, but I
didn't need it nine years before.

For whatever reason, the family physician has gone by the way-
side, not so much in the Mid-west, but on both Coasts. We've

never had a family physician since I've been here. And that's what's missing. That's the thing that caused health care to get off track to begin with. There isn't a guy that makes sure there's a real need before he says, "Yes, you need to go to an orthopedic surgeon or a cardiac guy or a neurosurgeon." The patient will just call the neurosurgeon directly and say, "I have a back problem. Will you see me?" If the guy has a hole in his schedule, of course he's going to see him. He's not going to turn him away.

The bad thing about the specialist, he trusts and he's used to getting his information based on certain diagnostic tests. If you're talking about a neurovascular guy, he's used to getting his best information from an arteriogram. So what's he going to do? He's going to order an arteriogram on everybody. Why? Because he figures why screw with all this other stuff? I'm just going to go here, and if it's negative, I do nothing. If it's positive I know exactly what I need to do. From his standpoint that's a perfect decision to make. It doesn't cost the doctor anything to do it. It's a good decision because they know they'll get the answer.

But on the other side, if they were triaged by the GP guy, he could say, "Well, let's do tests A and B before we jump to test Z." That's really more cost effective and it's better for the patient too. That's who the patient should go to first.

9

HOSPITALS—THE DONOR THAT KEEPS THE SYSTEM ALIVE

Anyone who has reviewed their bill after being discharged from the hospital must have asked themselves, "How can they charge this much? I could stay in a four-star hotel and pay less for a suite! If this isn't fraud and abuse, I don't know what is!" Are hospitals really making too much money, or are they just the easiest targets? When we talked to people working in hospitals, the consensus was that patients don't see the extent of the services provided, or the demands put on hospitals by patients and independent physicians.

Hospitals used to be a stable part of the community, but financial pressures have threatened many with closure and the long-term prognosis is bleak. In an effort to control costs, administrators have managed to wrench some control from physicians in some of the larger hospitals, but as in every other area of health care, caution must be exercised in order to insure continued quality of care.

A hospital is a losing proposition from the word "go." It always has been.

What three institutions in American society have the most in common? Hospitals, the military services and prisons.

These institutions have vividly contrasting purposes, but they employ the same methods, they all use the same techniques of dehumanizing their clients. They all use uniforms, general orders, absolute control of all activities of daily living, dictatorial authority, total domination and limits on personal freedom.

The process of events that reduce the patient's individuality, dignity and responsible self-assertion is called "hospitalization." The patients shift from an active, competitive world where he or she is aggressive and important, to a simplified world where even the smallest details of living—eating, defecating and physical position are dictated by strangers.

In one word, hospitalization is institutionalization. The big institutions such as the prisons, the military and hospitals are run by large numbers of people who employ the de-individualizing process to minimize their work load. Patients are stripped of their clothing, jewelry, identification papers and money. The person is assigned a uniform, a computer ID code and labeled as Dr. X's case number.

The doctor deals with disease and the patient's chart. Insurance companies, state licensing agencies, certification organizations and the rest of the bureaucracy are only concerned with the paperwork and an audit trail for the policy and procedures. There's never a concern for the human patient.

M ore and more small community hospitals are closing down. They cannot afford to stay open because of the lack of resources, the overutilization of medicine, and the drain on the system because of the indigent.

W e all know that there's overcapacity in the health-care system. Most of us in hospital administration don't want to say too much about it because it's going to mean hospitals will close, but we all know it. If you got rid of some of those hospitals you could save millions and millions of dollars that then could go toward wellness care.

T here will be a huge job loss, but it will be a job shift. We're seeing the unheard of thing of nurses being laid off now. For years and years and years there's been a nursing shortage. But it's happening because the system is already changing. It's moving from the highly personal, intensive acute-care setting into the primary care settings over a period of time.

There will always be a need for hospitals, but there will not be the need for hospitals that we have now by a long shot. That is going to happen whether the Clinton reform goes through or not. We are in a process now of reforming ourselves to be no longer just a hospital association. We need to be an association of integrated providers.

Our administrator recognizes the problem, our administrator is saying, "You know, to the extent that we are a delivery system, we can get patients to enroll so that they will be our enrollees instead of HMOs. Then, rather than us sitting and negotiating with an HMO who owns the enrollees—and we are competing with every other hospital in the area and they're trying to squeeze the lowest possible rate because they only need one of us—but if we can have some control over those lines, we can go to that HMO and say, 'We have five, ten, twenty-five thousand Medicare enrollees, or people who work for local companies have enrolled in our hospital medical integrated health plan.' " It puts you in a much better position to survive.

What hospitals are going to do is you'll find more of them banding together, especially the smaller ones, if they're going to survive.

Many hospitals are involved in outside private practices. In fact, almost every hospital that we see in southern California is involved in an outside private practice, either partially or totally. It's becoming more important. Because if they don't have people coming back in for surgery, if they don't have people referring for newborns and pediatrics, the hospital itself will die. They have to branch out to get revenue. What they do to make it better is they implement their quality standards at these outlying facilities. Our hospital is going out and getting these satellite practices because they figured if they don't do it somebody else is going to. That's a big push.

W e've put a big emphasis on customer relations and quality assurance in customer relations. People have a choice of either going here or there. We want them to come over to us. All the patients are given questionnaires when they leave the hospital, and I'm on staff to review anything that comes back from the patients.

You'd be surprised at the things people complain about the most. Number one is having to wait too long for a test, and that's anything over about fifteen minutes. We've got our standard at fifteen minutes. If a patient comes in and has to wait fifteen minutes, we have a supervisor out there telling them why they're waiting. If they have to wait any longer we continue to keep them updated. They want to know what's going on. The second thing is that a tech or a doctor or a receptionist was inconsiderate. Those are the two biggies that we get the most complaints on.

Anytime we get a negative, we'll call a patient, whatever it is, whether somebody had to wait fifteen minutes over their assigned time, or they sat out in the inpatient waiting area with their butt hanging out of their gown. Or even if the water level in the toilet was too high and a guy's testicles were in it—I'm serious about that one—we've called these people. We call them up, we talk to them, we let them air it out, and explain to them that it's not the norm. We're dealing with that sort of thing, and do try to assess those things.

The average patient isn't as concerned with cost as he is with waiting in line or wanting to be treated like a human being.

P eople don't want to travel any more than ten minutes for any type of service, I don't care if it's a hamburger or if it's picking up your cleaning, or health care. They won't travel thirty minutes to a hospital when they can travel ten minutes and get the same service. It may not be the same service, depending on the facility, but they think they're getting the service. Most people would pay the price there for the benefit of short distances.

I haven't been in an emergency room myself, even at the hospital where I work, and gotten out of there in less than three hours. I go to these Doc-in-the-boxes for runny noses and fingers that are sprained or broken and do them there. You can get good service and you get in and out a heck of a lot quicker.

When selling equipment to hospitals, there's not too many physicians that I've met that don't want the best quality. Until recently, say maybe three years ago, there was a concern that they got a good value. In other words, they wanted it for the cheapest amount of dollars, but they were willing to sacrifice money for quality. If they were convinced that one piece of equipment was better than another, if it had features that they absolutely had to have, or if the longevity of the equipment was excellent, they would go for it. What's happened now is those physicians have gone from the decision makers to only recommenders. The decision makers are now the business people, hospital administrators.

They've gotten involved, and in many cases detrimentally because they are absolutely cost conscious. What's most appalling to me is that most of the administration people are absolutely ignorant of the quality aspect. Although they talk about quality they will usually buy the lowest bid equipment that ends up in the long run costing more money or not being able to provide the service that it was actually originally intended to provide.

We found that the competition two or three years ago, was greater between hospitals. Now the competition is greater internally. By that I mean, administrators aren't as worried about what the hospital down the street or on the other side of town is doing, they're more worried about whether they can pay their bills and which managed care contract they're approved for and can get. Quality in decision making is becoming a secondary consideration.

Prior to about five years ago, most hospitals made it on their reputation. Today, people are becoming more conscious of cost, they're looking around, they're shopping. Especially the private payers, I'll get phone calls asking, "How much do you charge for an angiogram of the head? I'm calling other people too, and I'm going to find out."

There's really no standard in the industry to say how much you charge. I know how much it costs me, because I've sat down and figured . . . it takes this long, two techs and a nurse . . . an average angiogram costs $600 or $700 to do it, all things included. They're billed anywhere between $2,500 and $4,000 for it. Who sets those? There's nobody I know that sets those standards. Besides, you can charge whatever you want. You only get reimbursed so much anyway, especially Medicare and PPO contracts and HMOs. Basically, it's the individual's insurance company that's setting the price, not the hospital.

I t's turned around one hundred percent. The more tests you do on a patient nowadays, the more it costs you. The reimbursements on them are fixed. So if you get a hundred dollars for a patient that has "x" disease, and it costs you fifty to work it up, then you make fifty bucks. If it costs you a hundred and fifty bucks, you lose fifty bucks. So you don't care about the patients as much as you used to if you've got pressure on you from all sides to keep the cost of diagnosing and treatment under a hundred bucks.

H ospitals have always had a difficult time surviving. But now you have to be a four-star hotel if the patients are going to come. And at the same time, you're like a blood-let cow that's almost too weak to stand because everybody else thinks they deserve the health-care dollar first. If I was looking for an investment, I think hospitals would be the last choice where I'd put my money.

I think we're returning back to the hospital of the old days— without luxury amenities, without so many freebies for everybody, including doctors—just bare bones medical care.

Because community resources have become skimpier and skimpier, the hospital has become a social service agency. We have the homeless coming here for help now, not to the local Salvation Army. We have the battered women coming here for help, not going to the shelter. We have the person who has a doctor through the county, but maybe didn't have transportation to get there, take an ambulance here after hours. We're having the mental health patients, the psychiatric patients, come here because they can't get an appointment with the county mental health doctor. They show up here in the emergency room. The county and the state resources are not available after hours and weekends and nights. The shelters that are out there are full and the homeless have no place to go when it's cold and rainy. They show up at the hospital. The hospital has become the safe haven. The hospital has become the social agency.

We had a 77-year-old man show up yesterday, whose children were misusing his funds. He got tired of it, picked up and left, ended up out here and had no place to live. He tried staying on the street for a couple of days before he came to us and said, "I need help." We were able to get him some assistance. Seventy-seven years old and on the streets. That's what we're facing.

We're getting more and more indigent that we're treating. But you can do that more and more and more and more, until finally you drive yourself out of business. People look at hospitals and think that we're here to serve the public, but they don't understand that we have to make money to survive. When you're talking about that aspect, people think you're mercenary. Everything costs money to operate. And people are in this industry to make money too.

If you can't get paid for what you're doing . . . look at how many hospitals are closing their doors. Some hospitals are turning into these large trauma centers. People come in all shot-up, cut-up from gang warfare, run up $100,000 and then simply disappear. Or they don't pay for it. What are you going to do, take away their house because they can't pay their doctor bill?

W e very often are seeing more and more medically indigent coming into our hospital without money, without health insurance. They are very, very ill because they've gotten so ill in the community and have been unable to tap into any resources to take care of them. So now they are presenting to the emergency room at death's door. We are absolutely obligated to treat. We never turn anyone away.

Most times there is no reimbursement. In our county we still have what's available as our medically indigent adult program. L.A. County no longer has that program because it ran out of funding several years ago. The county will assist in paying for medical care, if the patient is stable for transfer to the county hospital and then continues to get their medical care through the county system. It's for those people that have no money and no insurance and can't pay for their health care and can't qualify for state aid.

We can never send someone away who's critically ill and not stable, and so hospitals everywhere are losing hundreds and thousands of dollars because people who started out with a common cold now have horrible illnesses that require long-term intensive care. Some of the issues that are raised in health care generally are, do we continue to treat and not get paid? At this hospital, because it's religious-owned we have a mission to help anyone who presents at our door and has a need. We don't turn people away. But I don't know if we will survive if those numbers continue to increase.

T he hospital board of directors is often made up of well-intentioned people selected for their financial or social position in the community. Frequently they are not informed on how the medical staff functions.

R egardless of ownership, hospitals have similar organizational structures. All medical staffs must develop and adopt bylaws and regulations to establish a framework for self-governance of medical staff activities and accountability to the governing body. Nonmedical people on the governing board are legally prohibited from practicing medicine, so the supervision of those activities must be delegated to the medical staff. When it comes to the medical staff's organization, there are two basic structures— departmentalized and nondepartmentalized. Both systems have an elected chief of staff and traditional officers of vice-chief, past-chief, chief-elect, treasurer and secretary. Both organizations have an executive committee and administrative housekeeping committees for medical records, utilization review, quality assurance, infection control, pharmaceutical, credentials, transfusions, nominating, ambulatory care, medical ethics, education, board liaison, and others as needed. The functions of these committees affect all specialty physicians on staff—family practice, internal medicine, surgery, obstetrics, pediatrics.

In departmentalized medical staffs, family practice doctors are in the Family Practice Department, all surgeons are in the Surgical Department, all internists are in the Internal Medicine Department, et cetera. Each specialty group elects its chairman who then becomes a member of the executive committee. Each department reviews physician applications and requests for privileges and makes recommendations to that executive committee. Each department is responsible for monitoring the physicians assigned to them.

In departmentalized medical staffs, there is a more judicious and conscientious review of the practice of medicine. Specialists protect their territory with a passion. If a member is not up to snuff, they will limit his activities or drive him away from the area.

Departmentalized medical staffs have at least one committee meeting a day. The hospital administrator is expected to attend as a nonvoting member. As the representative of the governing body, the chief executive officer will have major problems if he fails to attend all of the meetings.

Nondepartmentalized medical staffs are found in smaller hospitals. Committee assignments are made by the chief of staff who also appoints the respective committee chairmen. The number of committees can vary from one Committee of the Whole to as many committees as are found in the departmentalized medical staff. Supervision and granting of membership and privileges are much more lenient in the nondepartmentalized organization. For example, nonsurgeons vote on granting surgical privileges to themselves. The opportunity for fraud and abuse is far, far greater.

T he type of hospital ownership contributes to the lack of con-trol or encouragement of questionable medical practices. Community, nongovernment hospitals are divided into two broad categories: not-for-profit or for-profit.

You'll find less fraud and abuse in the not-for-profit hospitals; their objective is to have revenues exceed expenses enough to re-place equipment and buildings when necessary. Your best chances of quality care will be found in religiously affiliated hos-pitals. The Catholic hospitals, as a rule of thumb, are the most patient-centered of all hospitals; the more sisters that you see run-ning around, the higher the comfort level. Religious organiza-tions believe in the mission of helping the sick and you will often find medical ethics committees in those organizations.

Nonsectarian community hospitals do a fine job which varies with the size of the facility—the larger the hospital, the better are the chances of quality care. These hospitals also provide health education. Programs and services of these hospitals are not al-ways based on economics, but the unmet medical and social needs of the community. Not-for-profit hospitals generally have more staff, the level of personal care is higher.

As a rule, not-for-profits admit the more critically ill patients that are labor and equipment intensive. The shorter the hospital stay, the easier it is to balance the budget and to have an excess of revenues over expenses.

Then, you have the for-profit hospitals. There are investors to be satisfied. Most for-profit hospitals are part of large corpora-tions that have considerable business expertise. Their primary goal is to earn a profit. Often this colors the quality of patient care. These organizations enter into a more businesslike relation-ship with physicians, and if the doctor's greed gland can be acti-vated, it will be.

I 've been a hospital administrator for nearly forty years. If I were to tell a patient how to select a hospital, I'd suggest that as the first screening they look at the ownership—Who owns it? Then I'd prioritize them like this—first is best, last is the least recommended—religious, university affiliation, not-for-profit, for-profit, and HMO.

Then I'd check whether the hospital medical staff is departmentalized or nondepartmentalized. I would choose the departmentalized. In either case, check to see if the doctors are "board certified" or just "eligible." Being "eligible" means they have the training but have not taken the national examination. If they aren't, go down the street to another hospital. In that matter, if your doctor is not certified, delay the procedure until you get a second opinion from an academically qualified specialist.

There was this little fifty-bed hospital that had served a community for nearly thirty years. Surrounding communities had grown rapidly with modern medical services, shopping malls and regional businesses. The little town, controlled by elders, refused to see the changes until it was too late. Finally the hospital's directors realized that they would have to modernize the physical plant or go out of business, so the hospital began an aggressive program of purchasing neighboring property.

Before long they had contracted with an architect and had hired a bond consultant. The city fathers woke up in shock. If the hospital were to be built, it would be constructed on choice, center-of-the-town property. That meant one thing—they could never get a shopping center built in that prime location that would include their properties.

The city happened to have a redevelopment agency for renewal of a depressed business and residential area. Politics took over and the hospital was forced to surrender its properties and to accept a new hospital under terms that made it impossible to succeed. In the new 200-bed hospital, the city could move at any time to declare the hospital in default. The city fathers were in total control.

A miracle happened. The hospital was built and survived difficult obstacles. Slowly the activity increased, more doctors joined the staff and the reputation of the hospital dramatically improved.

For five years it was a struggle, then evidence of financial success started to appear.

Sounds like a happy ending, right? Well, a greedy physician saw a way to declare the hospital in default of the lease agreement, then purchase the hospital with a small group of friends. They tried to get the hospital administrator to be a party to the scheme, but he refused. Despite the administrator's refusal to participate, the doctor and his friends moved ahead with their plans. They contacted another hospital organization and negotiated the sale of the hospital.

Their plan was to have the hospital declared in default to the city, then purchase the hospital from the city and immediately resell it to the other hospital organization for a $10 million profit. They started their plan, and the hospital was declared in default of the lease. As a further example of the type of people we're talking about, the administrator was terminated on Christmas Eve.

Unfortunately for them, they had not counted on the hospital administrator's response. Together with the majority of the hospital's Board members, they moved the hospital into Chapter 11 bankruptcy. That prevented the immediate sale of the hospital and the unjust enrichment of the few unprincipled city elders.

The damage was already done though. The hospital's growth and financial solvency was destroyed. To this day, it has barely survived the event, and its reputation has been forever damaged.

I know of a 150-bed hospital located in a farming community that was originally owned and operated by a small religious order of women. It had been leased for management to a religious management company. The hospital prospered because it usually was filled to capacity.

Patient revenues were extraordinarily high, and the hospital controller soon became suspicious of the billing procedure. All bills were given to the administrator for approval of final diagnosis or the DRG, a Medicare billing designation that determines reimbursement regardless of the length of stay or services rendered. The administrator was creative. Boy, was he ever! He would change the DRG in order to maximize Medicare payment. The controller discovered the fraud and notified the corporation's regional vice president. The controller was told not to worry and was assured that the problem would be resolved. He waited and when nothing was done by the corporation VP, he reported the fraud to federal officials. The controller's employment was immediately terminated.

Eventually the hospital was found guilty of fraud and ordered to repay millions. How did the corporation respond? They leased it to another group who were to pay the penalties. The new group was ingenious in raiding the assets of the troubled hospital. They appointed the three owners of the new group to high-paying hospital positions, positions for which they never worked. They would charge the hospital for expensive meeting meals, $1,000 for three people. They bled the hospital of its receivables.

They never intended to pay the federal penalties, so they included a provision that if they failed in managing, the religious management corporation would have to repossess the hospital, including financial responsibility for all debts. That hospital is on the verge of bankruptcy.

Hospitals are the major economic cornerstone for the practice of medicine in the United States. Family practitioners and pediatricians could earn enough money to survive without hospitalizing patients or using the services provided by hospitals, but medical and surgical specialists would be out of business and on welfare if hospitals were not available.

Doctors control hospitals even though, in most cases, they don't have a personal financial investment in the facility. Can you imagine any other business that the customer can dictate the owner's policies, procedures and the selection and retention of employees? I've experienced firsthand how doctors can exercise financial blackmail over hospital management with impunity because they control the flow of patients and subsequent revenue.

Here's a simple example that is far too common. A physician was taken to a hospital's board of directors by the administrator for sexually harassing female employees. The official hearing found the

doctor guilty. The disciplinary action was that the board fired the
... doctor? No! They fired the administrator. Why? Because doctors
admit patients and order both inpatient and outpatient services. The
doctor produces revenue, the administrator doesn't.

M ost doctors, I suppose like any human being, will take
whatever the system provides. A few are clever entrepreneurs, and their greed is well hidden and disguised in the cloth of
"helping the patient" by controlling costs or convenience. They're
successful because the patient's primary concern is time spent,
not quality.

One example that I think is quite common these days is freestanding outpatient surgical centers. Physician investors see an
opportunity to siphon off hospital revenues by directing the patient to outpatient surgery investments. The total bill is usually
the same as one from a hospital outpatient surgery service, but
the hospital is cut entirely out of the revenue cycle.

What does the hospital get out of this? We get the uninsured
or minimally insured patient. We get the higher risk and more
expensive to treat surgical cases. What don't we get? Revenue
from simple and quick surgeries that help defray the cost of the
complicated cases. What do the physician-investors get? A hell of
a lot more income and less exposure and review of what they are
doing in their freestanding outpatient business. For all intents
and purposes, the doctors are not monitored for quality or necessity of care. Profits go up and up. All under the guise of taking
better care of their patients.

The same thing happens in other joint ventures such as freestanding imaging centers that contain all of the modern x-ray
technology. Beyond a doubt, such physician investments are a financial windfall for them. Referrals to such facilities increase
dramatically with a decrease of hospital-based activity. You see
profits increase dramatically for the physician-investors at the
same time that hospital losses grow.

F rom what I've seen, physicians, being in business for themselves, never hesitate to go into competition with hospitals

who provide the basic security for their careers. Politically, hospital management has never really been innovative in protecting its economic territory from the medical staff. Occasionally, we'll create joint ventures with physicians, but that's in order to retain a portion of the revenue stream needed to remain solvent. Sometimes these partnerships work. Usually they are only a temporary relief until the physician figures out another way to "share" a larger portion of the hospital's revenue.

I don't think people realize how dangerous these joint ventures become to the very life of financially stressed hospitals. Poor hospitals desperately need both outpatients and inpatients. When a doctor group offers to provide major diagnostic equipment like CAT scanners and MRI units to a financially weak hospital, the doctors dictate the terms of reimbursement. In one hospital where I worked, a group of seven orthopedic surgeons and radiologists provided a CAT scanner to the hospital. We were reimbursed a portion of the technician time but none of the utilities expenses. The hospital lost $30,000 a year on providing the service. The doctors made $250,000 to split among themselves. The chairman of the hospital board of directors was an attorney who just happened to have the physician investor group as a client. Guess what happened to the hospital administrator when he tried to renegotiate the lease terms with the physician investors.

Specialists depend almost entirely on hospitals for their survival. Anesthesiologists would be bankrupt without hospital surgical suites. All of the surgical specialists, orthopedic, thoracic, urological, neurosurgical, cardiovascular, obstetrics, gynecological, eye, cancer and ear, nose and throat could hardly function in a medical office surgery. There just wouldn't be the services of surgical and cardiac intensive care, highly trained nurses and technologists and millions of dollars of sophisticated equipment. Medical, nonsurgical doctors, would be handicapped without hospital services. Babies could be delivered at home, but where would the neonatal intensive care be provided for a sick newborn? Where would the obstetrician perform a lifesaving C-section?

S urgeons, regardless of specialty, earn money off the hospital by using the services, equipment and staff. Physicians who don't practice surgery take advantage of the freebies too! Cardiologists, pulmonary specialists, internal medical physicians with all of the sub-specialties, all suck at the udders of the hospital cows.

D octors pay nothing for the use of hospital services and equipment. If you as a singer want to record an album, you rent studio time. Surgeons pay absolutely nothing for use of the operating room, and then make unreasonable demands that if not fulfilled will cause him to take his patients elsewhere. When that happens, he tells the patient that the offending hospital can't provide the best service for his patients and convinces the patient that he is looking out for their welfare. Of course, the patient never really understands that the doctor's priority is his own interests first and the patient's next and the hospital's last.

R adiologists make exorbitant profits from the use of multi-million dollar hospital equipment for which they are not responsible to purchase, repair, replace, provide x-ray film, other supplies or technologist salaries. They seldom see a patient, and they charge an enormous amount for interpreting patient x-rays, most of which are routine. The films flip up and down on the x-ray view box and the doctor's words are recorded habitually on a dictating unit. The radiologist doesn't even pay for the transcription of his dictation. All of these services are free, so it's not unusual that a radiologist can earn over $500,000 a year with only minimum billing expenses for his portion of the charge for x-rays.

R adiologists are usually a contract service, but more and more are becoming part of the facility. In other words, they're a paid employee. Kaiser Permanente is a good example where the radiologists and surgeons all work for Kaiser. They're employees of the owners of the hospital and care facility. Same thing is happening with a lot of the other HMOs, the radiologists are not contracted. And it's not just the radiologists, the diagnostic services are not contracted.

The newer facilities are heading in that direction. It's the old established ones, where the contract was the way of doing it in the old days, that aren't. That may change. They're always looking at how they're going to save money, whether it will be financially beneficial. It's becoming more cost effective to have them on staff now.

P athologists have a real good game going. Years ago, it was established that hospital medical laboratories required a professional director. So, guess who is usually appointed to that position? A pathologist, although most of them haven't done a lab test since graduating from medical school. The price for this perk? Ten to fifteen percent of the gross revenue of the medical laboratory department. What do they do in return for huge contractual payments? Do they purchase, repair or replace equipment? No! Do they hire, pay and train employees? No! Do they stand any personal risk for failure of the lab? A little, and it's true they must have malpractice insurance. But the hospital is the deep pocket when it's time for the juries to make the awards.

T he hospital was in financial straits when I took the job. We couldn't afford to modernize our equipment. Being financially vulnerable, we were an easy mark.

Our mammography unit was about five years old, and there was much better equipment on the market. We had tried to upgrade the equipment, but even then, it didn't have all the conveniences like the automatic release of the breast after exposure.

Knowing that the hospital couldn't afford to buy one at the time, the radiologists demanded a new mammography machine. They refused to use the existing machine any more. However, they said they "weren't going to abandon the patients," so they decided to buy a new unit and install it in a building near the hospital. In essence, they had decided to go into competition with the hospital. The machine had already been ordered. They offered to have it installed in our x-ray department, but insisted that all the revenue had to go to their group. I recognize blackmail when I hear it, and I refused but was overruled by the board of directors. By the way, the chairman of the board just happened to be the attorney for the radiologists.

They worked this same deal with a CAT scan unit. Same group of radiologists plus some orthopods on that one. Both were lousy deals for the hospital, but great ones for the investing doctors. Of course, they overutilized the machines. They never thought it was a conflict of interest to order a $900 test for their patients. After all, they claimed they would have been negligent not to use the available equipment, especially if there were ever a malpractice case. They made a lot of money, while we lost a lot of money. So did the patients and insurance companies.

A hospital can be a very profitable operation, but only if it's owned by physicians. If revenue or occupancy goes down, the call goes out to increase utilization. It's a tap that can be turned on and off at will.

A group of doctors selected the hospital where they were on staff as a takeover target. It was a fairly new, attractive two-story facility, a little over two years old, nicely designed. The laymen owners had no desire to sell until business slowly came to a halt without explanation. For six months, the doctors used the services of other hospitals, but they kept just enough patients in the target hospital to prevent closure.

Finally, when there was just one patient left on the first floor and one more on the second, the doctors moved in to be the white knight for the owners. They offered an embarrassingly low price, and it was accepted. Within a few months, the place was making a healthy profit again.

Our hospital corporation purchased a 150-bed acute medical/surgical hospital from the original doctor owners. Negotiations had been tense and often hostile. The doctors valued the hospital far beyond its market value, but they'd heard rumors of other windfall sales and tried every way to increase their profits.

Part of the purchase price is called "goodwill," which translates into the doctors continuing to fully use the facility after they sell. The hospital had been running full with a tremendous profit, and we expected no significant change in utilization or profitability. To ensure our investment, a non-compete clause was included in the purchase agreement. This prevented the doctors from building another hospital in the area. We thought this was adequate protection for our investment.

The first inkling of trouble came with a report that an "anonymous" group had filed plans to construct a new hospital two miles away from the one we just purchased. Corporate staff members started to research the new project, but nothing tied in absolutely with that group of doctors.

Months went by and construction continued on the other hospital. Then the bombshell. We had retained key management people on assurances of employee loyalty and requests from the previous owners. The new hospital was due to open in ninety days, when all the key management employees submitted their resignations.

All hell broke loose. Elective surgeries were postponed. Morale of the uninvolved employees went to hell. The former owners became publicly hostile and vocal in their opposition to us. Revenue went to pot. Patient activity, both inpatient and outpatient, dramatically decreased. War had been declared and no prisoners were to be taken.

We had involved our attorneys from the first suspicions of something going wrong, but we had clever opponents. The doctors had invested in the names of others, like brothers-in-law, cousins, and maiden names of spouses. We went to court and won. We were awarded only a small judgment however. Our hospital survived poorly, was sold two times and finally closed fifteen years after our acquisition.

The result? Our investment was damaged. Duplicate hospital beds and services were created. Expenses increased, and the public had to pay a lot more for health care. The only ones to benefit were the doctors.

There was a little bit of satisfaction though. The leader of the bad guys had invested in the name of his partner who loved to fly and ski. Returning from a skiing vacation, he tried to land in a rainstorm and died. The widow inherited the leader's share of the new hospital, and she refused to let her husband's former partner gain ownership. The bastard had outsmarted himself.

10

LAWYERS AND INSURERS—THE NEW MEDICAL PRACTITIONERS

The general public and health-care professionals alike seem to believe that lawyers and the insurance companies leech the life-blood of the health-care industry and are the greatest reason for rising health-care costs. While we don't intend to exonerate them or act as their advocate, whenever blame is so easily assigned and the judgment is rendered with such emotion, it makes us wonder if the target is in fact a scapegoat, a way to avoid addressing the complexity of the problem. So to help broaden the discussion we have included stories that underscore the interrelatedness of the insurance industry, the legal profession and the health-care industry. For example, while the high costs of health care are irrevocably tied to the costs of malpractice insurance and litigation, at times the legal and the insurance industries perform the odd function of being the only watchdog on medicine. On the other side of the issue, and aside from the financial impact, their growing control of health care is indisputable. In many cases, the lawyer and insurance carrier are managing to practice medicine without a license—and are getting paid to do it.

There's too many attorneys hanging around making sure that insurance companies rule the world.

I f I ever go in the hospital I'm going to tell them that I'm an attorney. I think I would get better care.

W e have the legal system and the insurance companies. In health care, they're closely bound together. It's a vicious cycle, it seems to me. My brother-in-law, an OB-GYN, had to drop his OB because the cost was so high for insurance. He said it wasn't worth it to work that hard and then have to pay off such a huge insurance premium, so he just does GYN. I don't think it's any one system; those two systems together drive up costs.

I t just seems to me that in America, the insurance companies are making the big dollars on health care, and they're making it at our expense.

I n health-care terms, if we compared them to hospitals, mutuals are the not-for-profits, the others are in it to make a profit for investors. Those are the ones that people should be scrutinizing.

L et's start with a discussion on the concepts of insurance— what insurance is supposed to be and how it evolved generally, and then get into health insurance in particular.

Insurance, at least in the modern era, is really nothing more than a scheme to spread risk among people. I'll tell you the story of what may at least be part fact, part legend of an early example of insurance. Chinese traders on the Yangtze River came up with a technique that is a very rudimentary example of the spread of risk. Rather than loading all one person's goods onto one ship, they would divide them up so each of the barges held a portion of one another's goods. If one of the barges went down, a person only lost part, rather than their entire cargo.

Insurance then evolved through the Middle Ages and into the seventeenth and eighteenth century primarily for marine insurance, then into insurance for loss of life, and then liability. It wasn't really until the twentieth century that health insurance began to evolve.

Until this century, the economic consequences of ill health were not like they are today, because we didn't have the technology, we didn't have the resources available for which people can spend money. Life expectancies were much shorter and there were not prolonged periods of hospitalization or convalescence. Particularly during the civil war and into the early decades of this century, we saw a lot of breakthroughs that led to longer periods of care and hospitals became a place for true treatment, rather than just a convenient place to die. The cost of hospital care began to be a concern, and people began looking for ways to finance the care via some type of insurance or prepaid mechanism.

The original Kaiser plan was devised by Henry Kaiser as a means of providing care, not as insurance. When he was building projects in remote areas, he hired physicians to go with the employees. Eventually that was expanded to cover the families, and Kaiser recognized that this could be extended beyond his own employees. Ross Loos was also an early example, but his was prepaid care; that is, pay a premium and receive the assurance of services available for those membership dues. During the 1930s, a number of hospitals devised similar capitated plans. You had the Depression going on, and people were certainly not able to afford the cost of hospitalization, but could afford the fifty cents or dollar membership dues that would entitle them to coverage.

With the advent of the second world war, companies had to freeze wages by order of the government, but employers still had a very critical need for workers. The wage/price controls did not extend to so-called fringe benefits, so to attract and retain employees, employers began a more widespread practice of providing health care and other benefits in lieu of wage increases. At about this time the first health insurance policy was written for a labor union, and in 1948 the Taft-Hartley Act said that benefits were a legitimate item for negotiation between labor and management.

Typically this hospital and surgical coverage would provide thirty days of hospital care—primarily for food and room and the limited services that the hospital was able to provide. It was really to cover the cost of your hospital stay. Compared with today, there were not too many things that would generate costs. Doctor bills and drug bills were relatively low. You either recovered fairly quickly or you died.

In the 1950s, before the discovery of a vaccine, polio was a real threat, resulting in long-term confinement at very great expense. Insurance companies began developing so-called "Dread Disease" or "Polio" policies to supplement the basic hospital or surgical plan. Then came the recognition that people could incur expensive extended care, not just from dread disease, but from other types of long-term illnesses as well, so major medical insurance evolved as a supplement to the basic hospital and surgical policies. Major medical introduced the concept of the "deductible."

Health insurance became catastrophic coverage for two reasons. Number one, as care became more complicated, costs began surpassing the daily dollar limits or duration limits—I've cited thirty days—under those policies. Polio is a prime example for the second reason. There were specialized clinics set up for treatment of people with polio—we might call them sanitariums. Sanitariums could charge far less than hospitals, yet the people had no insurance for them because their policies were limited to accredited hospitals.

In the late fifties, early sixties, we also began to see the beginnings of outpatient therapy. People would go to the hospital not necessarily to be kept overnight but to use the facilities that were there. But the insurance was really inpatient insurance, so insurance became catastrophic in the sense that there it began to include other treatment modalities not covered by the typical policy. As major medical insurance became more and more popular, and most employer plans provided a major medical type of benefit.

In 1966 came the passage of Medicare which created a tremendous increase in demand for health-care services. Prior to Medicare, for the most part the elderly had no health coverage. A few had retiree coverage through their employers or union plans, but it was not that common. People relied on their employer's coverage while they were working, and when they retired they had to finance health care out of personal savings. Medicare was referred to as a "credit card" system which people over sixty-five could take to any doctor and get whatever services the doctor attested that they needed. The government, through Medicare, was really a fairly adequate provider of coverage, at least in the early days. Hospitalization (Part A Plan) was provided free to anybody who was covered under Social Security. The professional piece (Part B Supplementary Plan) has always been subject to a premium—initially was a couple of dollars a month, now it's around forty-dollars.

The insurance companies saw this market that was previously financing the cost of care itself, but now had the federal government picking up 70 to 80 percent of the cost of care, and recognized that the dollars these people would have spent anyway, they would be interested in spending to supplement what the government was doing. Prescription drugs and private duty nursing are the two most significant areas not covered by Medicare. The insurance companies began selling policies to cover these, and in addition, policies to cover all or part of the first day of hospitalization, which Part A didn't cover, or hospitalization extending beyond ninety days.

Then by the mid-to-late seventies, Medicare was limiting more and more the amount that it would pay for physicians. It might, for example, pay $400 on an appendectomy, even though the average cost of the surgeon might be $600. The individual then had that out-of-pocket difference, so "Medi-Gap" policies began to proliferate. And while it's important to have all three policies, unfortunately a lot of older people were sold coverage that was redundant—they didn't really understand what they had or what they needed. About three years ago the government passed some fairly stringent "Medi-Gap" laws and there's now a national set of standards and benefit criteria.

I can remember back in the early seventies, when the daily costs of a hospital room was still only running about $150 a day, $50 for the room and an additional $50 for the ancillary services. When we compare that with the costs of, typically, $800 to $1,000 per day that are common, it's amazing. It's really amazing.

Health insurance is often looked at as one of the reasons that contributed to it. I would contend that while it did contribute, it was really reacting to a demand of the public for protection against these events, fueled really by employers who were willing to provide the coverage in lieu of wages. And in effect, insurance insulated a lot of individuals from the true costs of their care. Using the credit card analogy, when they have little personal stake in paying the premiums, it was easy for them to simply demand more coverage. When you add to it the significant growth in federal entitlement programs during the sixties and seventies, it's easy to see how the concept of entitlement began to grow. People felt that access to health insurance as a funding mechanism was a right to which they were entitled and that somebody, somewhere was going to pay for it. I don't think you can blame the insurance industry alone for this.

The costs in the early seventies, relatively low by today's standards, were already beginning to rise at a fairly rapid pace, leading to a lot of concern about the ability of the employers and the ability of the country in general to pay. In 1973 the HMO Act was signed by President Nixon. Recognizing the value of the Kaiser-type system, it made government money available for organizations to create HMOs. It also gave them a built-in market because it gave federally qualified HMOs the right to go out and mandate that their plans be offered to employers with twenty-five or more people in a given service area.

There are probably three to four hundred HMOs around this country. They have tended to be regional in scope, but there is a new trend towards creating HMOs that are national in scope, primarily to benefit the very large employer whose work force is not concentrated in a single city.

HMO coverage was typically better than that found under the indemnity insurance plan of the time, because it often had no front-end deductible and it tended to cover a larger range of items. The disadvantage was that these plans attracted younger families, whose average health-care costs were probably less than the population as a whole. The costs of indemnity insurance, the traditional major medical type of plan, tended to rise even faster than it might have otherwise because it lost the leveling influence of these younger, healthier people. So the insurance industry came up with the concept of a PPO, or a Preferred Provider Organization. This allowed insurance companies to reduce their rates on the basis that there are preferred provider networks in place;

the insurance company would negotiate with these for reduction in rates.

Up until that point, large employers or the government were looking for insurance companies to reduce their costs by focusing on the administrative expenses—an average of eight to twelve percent of premium, which included the costs for processing claims, investigating claims, cutting the checks, and the computer systems, et cetera. With the introduction of the PPOs, the focus now turned to the cost of the claim itself, saying, "Let's not allow a person to simply get medical care at the prevailing rate, let's negotiate a lower rate with some doctors and hospitals in return for the promise that we'll channel more business their way."

The PPOs really began to grow in the early 1980s, and by the end of that decade you had HMOs holding probably a thirty-five percent market share, PPOs probably a fifty percent share, and traditional insurance, in which you could go to any doctor of your choice and have the entire bill, or eighty percent of it, paid in full, a dwindling percentage.

In the late seventies and early eighties, employers were finding their health-care costs on average rising twenty, twenty-five, and in some cases thirty percent per year. They felt they had no control over those costs—wages they had control over. But the health-care component, the "fringe benefit," continued to soar.

Fringes in total began to rise to thirty, thirty-five and in some industries close to forty percent of payroll. Not all of that was health care of course—you had vacations, the employer's contributions to Social Security, and other mandated benefits. But health care was easily the fastest-growing segment, and employers became very frustrated, so they started pressuring the insurance companies to do something. Some employers took steps like saying, "We'll put a one hundred, two hundred, or three hundred dollar limit per day in the plan. We'll limit what we pay for a doctor to 'x' dollars."

The problem with that is, if it's a $200 daily limit and hospitalization is $300, all the employer has done is cost-shifted the difference to you. You're paying it out of your wages. The employer can say, "We just can't pay increases without limit. You have to pay some of this risk yourself." But from a competitive standpoint, it was very difficult to look employees in the eye and say, "Here's why we're giving you what has become an inadequate plan."

Employers needed a means to affect the costs, and that's one of the reasons that initially HMOs, then later the PPOs, became popular. They found that they could negotiate lower costs—particularly very large companies in the Mid-west, in towns where one employer is dominant. In some of these factory towns, that one employer really had a lot of clout with local doctors and hospitals. He could negotiate fees in which they couldn't increase more than a fixed percent. He was able to put pressure on them and say, "If you don't agree to this contract, I'll find somebody else, and direct my employees there."

Another way large employers tried to contain costs was with a third-party intermediary, a go-between who adjudicates the claims process. For example, you often hear the term "fiscal intermediaries," which are used by Medicare. If you are covered by Medicare, you don't submit your bill to the federal government, you submit your bill to one of the insurance companies as a fiscal intermediary in your area.

Large employers, historically, bought coverage through insurance companies, meaning the insurance companies established a rate per person, the employer paid that rate and out of the pool that the insurance company collected from the employer, it would pay claims. Sometimes the larger employers could negotiate dividends or refunds of unused monies; certainly, the larger employer could negotiate that next year's rates would be set largely on the basis of past experience.

Beginning with 3M in 1970, the large employers went to the insurance companies and said, "We want you to just act as a service bureau for us. We'll pay you an administrative fee, but we're not going to pay you a premium every month. You just administer the plan, and when it's time to pay the bills, you let me know the amount of checks you're ready to issue, and we'll give you the money that you need to cover those claims." There, the insurance company is acting as a third-party intermediary (Third Party Administrator). It's very confusing because it's still the same insurance company using the same personnel, but typically the check they issue for the claim will have the employer's name on it and say something like, administered by the Equitable Life Assurance Society.

In addition to the cashflow advantage, the employer can save two to three percent of the annual premium because those transactions are not subject to state premium taxes, which money paid to an insurance company would be. Nor are they subject to the profit and risk charges that an insurance company would make. So you typically get a two to three percent savings in addition to whatever you save from the cashflow, of not having to put your premium up front every month.

While large employers have gained control in some areas, they are losing some in others. Originally, a lot of the rating was based on a so-called "community rated" concept. The insurance company comes in and says, "OK, for people of this average age in this area, we'll charge this rate." As the popularity of employer-driven group insurance increased and it became a more competitive marketplace, insurance companies recognized that if they could identify the good risks, those groups of people who were likely to have lower claims, and get those groups enrolled, then they'd make more money because they'd spend less on the claim dollars.

A whole variety of rating systems began to evolve. Some insurance companies recognized that some ethnic groups, just by virtue of their culture tend to use insurance or doctors far less frequently. In organizations that had a predominance of young healthy employees, banks or schools, particularly in the days when maternity was not covered, insurance companies found that the average costs for a teacher group or a bank with a high female population, were far less than the average cost of a manufacturing population of 45- to 50-year-old males.

So they began a whole new series of experience rating formulas and the larger employers began demanding more accountability from the insurance companies on the wellness, if you will, of their work force. Some employers, even in the early days, would screen their own employees to make sure that they were hiring a healthy work force and their thinking was, shouldn't we get some benefit of that from our insurance company? So insurance companies were being pressured to give money back for good ratings, either as dividends or in the form of lower rates next year. Employers began to become more and more sensitive about their costs of care.

This shift from a community rating to a rating for an employer, even an employer with several thousand employees, means you're now spreading the risk of catastrophic care for that employer's work force among a much smaller base than you would have if it was spread throughout the entire community. Employers began to be very sensitive about catastrophic diseases like AIDS; this has gotten a lot of publicity because of the efforts of some employers to limit their liability for AIDS.

Introduction of preexisting condition exclusions by employers was an effort to eliminate their need to provide care for people who came to work with an existing medical problem. The termination of coverage immediately following employment, and that could include termination of employment because of medical conditions, became very common and led to significant hardships on people. That led to pressure from the government to prohibit employers from just cutting off coverage—they had to provide some means for those employees to have continued coverage at the time that they most need it. One of the things that national health care does is to try to push us back to a form of a more community rating. Under the Clinton plan, except for the very largest employers where the threshold is 5,000 employees, rates are going to be set on a community-rated basis, so that employers can't benefit from the good health of their own population. It's going to be blended among a larger group.

Many people believe that the insurance companies are making too much money on health insurance. It certainly varies from company to company, but insurance companies tend to make far more money off of investments than the underwriting profits, which is the premium revenue minus the cost of claims and the cost of administration. At best, that's been one or two percent; for some insurance companies it's been negative for several years. The missing piece in that is the reserves they hold. With the exception of the two to three months' reserve, the money is turned over fairly quickly and paid back out in claims. You don't have long periods of time in which to accumulate investment returns like you do with life insurance, or even disability insurance, where they hold your premiums for long periods of time. Insurance companies don't make a lot of money on health insurance. A lot of them stay in the health-care marketplace for one reason only: to have the product available. They want their agents to be able to sell a complete portfolio that would fit the needs of the individual or small business owner.

What are the insurance companies doing in reaction to the trends in health-care coverage? Some of them have gotten out of the health-care business—they've withdrawn, or they've sold that block of their business to some other insurance company. Others have tried to create incentives for people to assume a greater share of the risk—you'll find insurance companies that will give discounts for nonsmokers, or discounts to some employers who have various types of wellness plans in their companies.

In the indemnity plans, where insurance companies pay the doctors and hospitals when there are services to be rendered, they're constantly battling the doctors and the hospitals; challenging the necessity of the care, the duration of hospitalization, the necessity of the surgery, looking for use of generic drugs rather than brand name drugs, all in an effort to hold down their claims costs.

On the HMO side, some of the insurance companies are finding ways to attract lower-cost populations, pointing out to doctors and hospitals that because the insurance company is screening the patients for small employers with a short health statement [a questionnaire determining risk factors], the doctor's going to be dealing with a healthier class, and therefore, he can afford to take a lesser monthly capitation rate to treat this class of patient because it's not going to involve as much of his time. The resources needed will not be as great as for an average population or a population where there would be no exclusions on preexisting conditions.

You've got the best known trade association for insurance companies, the Health Insurance Association of America, taking a very aggressive stand, and generating some ire from Hillary over it, trying to educate people to what it sees as some of the underlying facts of the Clinton legislation that are not obvious in their descriptions. The HIAA is lobbying hard for a plan that will still give them a very active role in sale and administration and in the ability to set prices. Their biggest concern is that their prices are going to be squeezed by some type of global budgeting process. They feel that they're going to be squeezed into providing a specified level of benefit and will not be able to generate the revenue that they need to pay for that.

Insurance companies are in business to make money. A lot of people don't understand that concept. They're not in business to feel sorry for someone who has an accident and requires medical attention. They are not charitable organizations. That's where the insurance companies have really snowed the public.

Oftentimes when you're enrolled in a specific insurance plan, your employer makes the choice. A lot of folks come in and they want to trade here but they can't because they've just been enrolled by their employer in a new health plan and the health plan has a limited list of providers. The patient should decide which physician he's going to see, not an insurance bureaucrat, not an employer.

Insurance companies offer these "take it or leave it" contracts to providers. There is no negotiation. You're given a piece of paper; either you sign it or you don't. If you don't, you're not in. It's that simple. If you sign it, you have turned over virtual control of your business to the insurance industry. They now will determine your price.

This is a real troublesome issue, when you have the insurance industry controlling the providers on the one hand, and they're controlling the patients on the other, what do we have?

Health insurance is an anomaly in the insurance industry. Every other kind of insurance you buy is catastrophic. It doesn't pay the maintenance costs. Normally, your fire insurance doesn't pay to replace your roof with fire resistant material or clean up the dead brush around your house. Your life insurance doesn't pay you if you have financial problems during your lifetime. Your property insurance doesn't cover the costs of improvements or repairs on your building. Why is health insurance expected to pay for every little expense regarding your health?

M y mother got pancreatic cancer. My father and I took care of her. We brought her home to care for her because that was the bottom line for Medicare—six days. If you're not cured in six days, you're out on the street. They'll put you out and bring you back in, but you have to be out three days. So the family takes them home to care for them.

Well we had taken care of her for four months and four days, and the pharmaceutical bill was $4,000. Medicare wouldn't pay it because a registered nurse wasn't administering the medications. That's how they got by without paying. And my mother's supplemental insurance said, "We only pay eighty percent of the twenty percent that Medicare doesn't pay." But Medicare didn't pay anything, so they refused to pay anything too, and my father got stuck with a bill for $4,000.

O ne of the problems is, speaking more from what I've heard from physicians, why should an insurance claims adjuster, somebody with a high school education, be telling physicians what to do, how to manage the case? I think there's a lot of validity to that.

W e decide who to pay, what to pay, and how much to pay. The doctor will fill out a form and the treatments will start and when the bills come in, they're referred over to a medical evaluating facility and they'll review the bills and what we're being charged for, whatever criteria they have, they'll adjust the bills and say, "We recommend you pay this." If we're being charged $100, they may say, "That's unreasonable. Pay them $50." I don't know what their criteria are, but that's how we determine how much to pay.

When someone came in the hospital for an ulcer, first they would do a gall bladder. Then they would do a barium enema. Then the next day they'd do a GI series and then a small bowel. They would do thousands of dollars in examinations to find out that the guy had a peptic ulcer, which the doctor may have used as his admitting diagnosis. So after days in the hospital, going through all these examinations, the doctor prescribes some ulcer medicine and sends him home, which is what he should have done from his office in the first place.

What the insurance companies are doing is saying, "You need to have a clear-cut diagnosis. If you take this patient in the hospital for a hangnail on his big toe, you're not going to x-ray his head and his stomach and his small bowel and his shoulder. We're not going to pay for it."

If you have auto insurance, that's to protect you if you're in a severe accident. They don't pay if you get a flat tire, auto insurance is not involved in those small things. They don't replace your windshield wipers or your motor oil or your spark plugs. They don't pay for your gasoline. What has happened in health-care insurance is they now want to do all of the above. Why? Because for every single transaction that they're involved in, they can charge a fee. [These fees are plan administration costs that come out of the premiums.]

Let's say you're a patient and you need a prescription filled. You come to me and you have an insurance plan. Say it's a $10 prescription. Now you can pay me the $10, but you have a plan that's only going to cost you $2. So you give me $2 and I bill the insurance company for the other and they get a fee. Why should we pay them to be in the middle of a $10 transaction? It doesn't make any sense, but that's exactly what the insurance companies have done. The more transactions they're involved in, the more money they make.

I'm going to show you how they turned a $6 prescription into $16. It's magic. Several years ago I had a fellow come in from the dentist here with a prescription for acetaminophen with codeine. My price was $6.25. Well, his insurance company would only allow me $5.85. This wasn't so bad, so we accepted it. I filled the prescription, he gave me his $2, and I billed his insurance company.

For processing the claim, they get five bucks. So you add their five bucks to my $5.85, that's $10.85. But, they rejected it. I got what was called a turn-around. I had to do it again. I checked my copy and they had made the mistake. I suspect they make a lot of mistakes on purpose. I resubmitted the claim and finally I got paid. OK. That $6.25 prescription cost $16. And here's how.

I got my $5.85. They got their $5 processing fee for processing it the first time, then they got another $5 for processing the turn-around document. The insurance company gets $10 and all they do is shuffle paper. I get $5.85, which includes the cost of the drug and all my other costs. My profit was about three bucks. The insurance company's profit is ten and what should have cost $6 costs $16.

That's how it got so out of hand. The insurance companies are like the 300-pound gorillas on the back of health-care providers. That's just one example and there are thousands of them just like that.

W hen I was a claims manager, every November and December, we'd go through all of our cases for the entire year, and make a file of every case that was still pending, all our open files. Most files would take five years of litigation, so we always had a lot of files that were still open.

With each of these open files, our orders were to calculate the reserve—the amount that you thought they will settle for. In the case of, say, an eye poked out. You'll reserve $500,000, even though you know damn well you can settle for a $100,000. You'll reserve high because if you reserve low and you're paying out more than your reserve, you're going to get fired.

So each November of every year, we were told to review our file and raise our reserve. They would normally say, double it. So in the case where someone's lost an eye, that five hundred thousand for the injury, you'd reserve it to a million. Why? That amount of money would then go into reserve for claim payments. It's reserved and not considered income, so it's nontaxable.

I 'm a defense attorney for a workers comp insurance company. I'm also a medical doctor. Maybe it's because I would expect the physicians to have a little higher ethical standards, but the worst fraud I've seen is by medical groups that are set up just to milk the workers compensation system. Some of it is just blatant fraud, creating claimants who do not exist or who are dead. Or, what is much more common is just exaggerating everything to the hilt. If you walked in there, they'd find six things wrong with you that you had no idea you had, and no one else would find wrong with you either. Then they refer—I compare it to an octopus— they refer to every specialty they can think of and get $1,000 to $2,000 for each consult in each specialty.

Both the state and federal governments have gone after them, but it's difficult to nail them with fraud because there's so much discretion involved in these things. If they handle one legitimate case out of a hundred that gives them some credibility. And it's probably more than one out of a hundred.

A s an insurance claims adjuster, I guess what really irritates me is the fraud involved. It ends up being seen in the premiums that we all pay. We're all being run out of business because of it. A lot of people are getting away with it. Even if we suspect fraud, a lot of times it's more cost effective just to pay the claim than to try and fight it in the courts.

There are those doctors that we know are involved in insurance fraud, but we still have to proceed with each individual claim as though it was legitimate. The burden of proof is on us. We can't just shut them down, because there's always legitimate claims intermixed with the fraudulent ones. Most could be fraud, but some aren't. These people know the system and how to work it.

B ring the fees more in line with what's standard for traditional medical care. It's not unusual for a specialist—an orthope-

dist, or a psychiatrist, or a neurologist—to get somewhere between $1,200 and $2,000 for a workers comp evaluation. Supposedly this takes four to eight hours' work, in reality, they may have
only spent one hour because they would turn out several patients
a day.

I think an enlightened view would be that if someone has an
injury, the best thing to do is get that person treated and back
to work, not increase their stress level and exacerbate their physical condition. Try to weed out the ones that are fraudulent, but
also try to be careful that all the ones that are legitimate are taken
care of. That's the way the system is set up, and it should operate
that way. But people's individual ideologies and biases come into
play. There are people on one side that think everybody is legitimate and everybody should collect if they feel they're injured.
And then there are others who feel that nobody should collect,
that everybody is fraudulent.

I know of a medical center that has a program where when
they identify malpractice as having occurred, they actually approach the patient and tell them what has happened, and offer
them whatever they feel is an appropriate response, from free
treatment to compensation. As of a few years ago they'd only had
two cases that actually went to trial. They're unusual in that but
they've probably saved themselves a good deal of money in the
process, in addition to having a more humane approach. I'm sure
they're not unique, but are probably the exception rather than
the rule.

The insurance carrier may be more prudent to settle for a
small amount of money on a claim that has questionable
merit, than to spend twice that amount on their attorneys and the
system to fight it. Which encourages more claims. So it's a Catch-
22 situation.

The insurance companies go in cycles. "We are not going to
pay any more nonmeritorious claims. It's going to be dollars for
defense and not a penny for tribute. We're going to go all the
way." It's kind of refreshing when that happens because now I

know how to prepare the case and get ready for trial. On the other hand when they're waffling, when you've prepared and you're ready to go and you know that you've got an excellent chance of beating it, and then at the last moment they come up with some large amount of money. It makes me wonder. Why are they paying me $30,000 or $40,000 to get this ready for trial and now coming up with $150,000? Why didn't they come up with $150,000 months ago? Those are the things that cause insurance premiums to go up, too.

We can tell what the jury verdicts are in malpractice, but we can't tell what the settlements are.

Down at the dead center of this issue of malpractice is a sleeping monster, and that's the insurance company. The doctors will tell you that they have to charge higher prices because of their higher malpractice premiums, and the insurance companies have such a stranglehold they can charge whatever they want. I've had the governor of California order the Commissioner of Insurance to ask the insurance companies, "What are your premiums for malpractice for the last year?" The insurance companies told the Commissioner, "Go to hell. We won't give it to you."

As the years go on, you see the malpractice verdicts going higher and higher. The defense lawyers representing the insurance companies are the ones who will deliberately put a case to trial. A lot of times it'll be a case where they should have settled it. But they're getting paid by the day, so they fight the cases real hard. That's why, when they fight a case, and the jury says, "Hey, wait a minute. This doctor really did screw up. He killed this person," the verdicts go clear off the wall.

Then the lawyers representing the insurance company release those big verdicts to the newspaper. Within a day or two every doctor has read it. Then the insurance company raises its premiums because "those crooked lawyers got all this money off this case." In reality, the insurance company is saying, here's our opportunity to stick the knife in.

You can take every single malpractice case and settle it for cheaper than you can try it. But bear in mind the insurance company wins two-thirds of the cases. The others are runaway verdicts. In spite of that, the insurance companies recoup their losses and actually increase their revenues in raising their rates, more than they ever pay out in big verdicts.

The insurance companies are the real beneficiaries of caps on verdicts. It's not the doctors, they're going to be paying higher premiums no matter what. It's definitely not the patients, they're innocent victims who may not be justly compensated. It's the insurance companies that have their liability limited. Just try to find out sometimes what they pay through lobbyists in state capitals, or in Washington, D.C.

If you could get a case book, you could track all of the malpractice verdicts and settlements. These statistics would tell a tremendous story. The problem is, you can't.

Now let's say, just for a number, we discover the total verdicts are four hundred million in our state. That's the number I came up with one year. Some would figure, "Hey that's total verdicts, four hundred million." Then a little light flashes. Wait a minute, how much went to the bank of the $400 million that the juries said insurance companies owed to the plaintiffs? You would expect that the insurance companies wrote checks for $400 million and that's it. Right? Wrong.

There's what they call appeal. I calculated that in one year, $16 million went to the bank out of $400 million. What's happening in effect is the insurance companies are saying, "Screw you! We don't care what the verdicts are. We don't care what your laws are in this state or anywhere in the country. We're not going to pay it."

That just happened the other day on a medical malpractice case. The first verdict went through at two-and-a-half million. The insurance company refused to pay it, so it went up on appeal, they were granted a new trial. The second time, it went for seven-and-a-half million. I called the attorney and said, "Hey, great, you got seven and a half million the second time around." He said, "We settled the case for four million."

People don't know it, but what you're awarded in verdicts isn't necessarily what the insurance company actually pays. People are getting what the insurance company feels like giving them. In this case, they felt like giving them four million in the face of two and seven. And that's only because they were afraid that if it went to trial again it would be fifty million.

I f you're a doctor and a malpractice case settles, it's because you said you were wrong. So don't talk to me about innocence if you've already admitted you're wrong.

A lot of attorneys have gone into the legal profession with pretty high ideals. Many of them come into the legal profession as liberals. Most social-service kind of mentalities tend to be liberal. It's not a very difficult jump for those people thinking in that direction to believe that any person injured should be taken care of regardless of fault, regardless of circumstances. That's not an altogether bad concept. But then the next step is, the insurance companies have the money so I'm going to go get it for them.

Then after the attorney has been in this business for five or ten years some get very cynical and they're in it to make money. Most attorneys really aren't in the profession to make money. It happens because of the way it's built. Many lawyers are perceived as predatory and carnivorous, and much in the nature of a vulture, sitting on the fence ready to devour the carcass before it's even stopped quivering. We have that image because we are usually called on only when there's a lot of problems, big problems.

A physician in Michigan, an OB-GYN who delivers babies, recently responded to a national magazine on a story they had done about the high cost of health care. His comment was something like this. "There's an attorney in my state who makes in excess of seven million dollars a year in suing strictly OB-GYNs. I would have to work thirty years to make that much money. If you want to address the high cost of insurance, let's start with this. It is outrageous that one attorney is making that kind of money simply by suing doctors like they're infallible."

That's hard to gauge, public opinion towards lawyers and malpractice. There have been a number of studies that show that people like their individual attorney but hold the profession in quite low regard. It's unfortunate. Obviously, there's an element of the profession that are bottom dwellers. But isn't that true of every profession? Physicians, the media and the insurance companies are big culprits in promoting this. It keeps the spotlight off these other groups.

It's just a stupid circle. Attorneys love to get those big cases because they can bill the heck out of them. And the doctor, his ego is at stake, so he says, "Don't you pay this claim."

Physicians in most places always strive for quality. I don't think that I've worked for too many that don't try to have the best possible equipment to give them the best diagnosis, to make their job the easiest to do. But the litigation aspect is always sitting above everybody like this scrooge cloud. Everybody talks about quality, but the only reason they talk about quality so much is because they're worried about getting their butts sued off by somebody.

Because we live in such a sue-happy society, doctors are ordering tests that probably are not necessary. They know if they don't, they're opening themselves up to major liability. What if this is the time that the belly pain isn't just a stomachache or diarrhea from eating something bad? What if this is the time when someone's got something serious going on inside? Most of the time, doctors can pick up on things without doing a battery of tests, but because there's such a craze of "I'll sue you," they have no choice.

Even with the welfare recipients. A lot of them say, "If you don't give me the right care, I'll sue you." They've got free medical care, but if they don't get treated the way they want to, they're threatening to take you to court. You're looking at them going, this is ludicrous.

A lot of physicians are scared to death of malpractice suits. The physicians that could treat the common cold, now say, "I think you have sinusitis. You need to go down to the radiologist and have your sinuses x-rayed." And then they send you over to an ENT—ear, nose and throat—guy. They didn't used to do that. They would treat it the best that they could, and probably succeed, but the fear of malpractice has convinced them of the advantages of referrals. You still get paid, but you're putting a big chunk of the malpractice liability on someone else's shoulders.

I 'm a trial attorney handling defense work mainly for insurance carriers. It's very much a PYA (protect your ass) attitude now. It's not unusual for an anesthesiologist or a surgeon to pay $80,000 to $100,000 a year premium for insurance. That's a staggering sum of money.

Until you get away from the concern that the doctors are targets—they've got the money therefore let's go get it—and can reduce those premiums on the malpractice coverage to within a reasonable area, I don't think you're going to get a handle on this. As long as they feel they have to protect themselves in order to treat a patient. They're going to overtreat. They're going to overprescribe. That has been built into the system in the last fifteen or twenty years.

B inding arbitration is the answer. Arbitration as it is now is not binding. When a mistake is made, they should immediately sit down and try to establish the facts of the case. An arbitration panel should be selected, composed of objective third-party medical professionals—not lawyers, and not insurance companies. They sit down and call in everyone related to the case and record it all. They should ask, "Now, doctor what happened?"

They don't need to take any bullshit from anybody, they just get right to the center issue.

Once the facts are gathered, then, they put their insurance company on notice. No one tampers with the testimony. The insurance company can read it, but so can anybody else. You wouldn't have to go through lawsuits. You wouldn't have to put a patient and their family through agony for five and a half years before trial.

Then, you could address the cause of the problem: Why did it happen? How can we prevent it from happening again? Was this a reasonable mistake on the physician's part, or does he have a history of blunders? In other words, the process doesn't end just with financial compensation to the one who's been injured. It takes steps to prevent another person from suffering in a similar way.

I'd go to arbitration. There are so many nuisance suits that are brought just because somebody is angry, not necessarily because they have a good suit. They're just hoping you won't fight it, the malpractice insurance company will just write a check.

Binding arbitration will not, cannot, solve this problem because binding arbitration is also adversarial. Arbitration would make law more efficient, but the adversarial aspect of it wouldn't change.

What it will do is it will eliminate some of the congestion in the courts so we have room for the drug heads and the criminals. But it's just moving the venue.

Piecemeal tort reform is not going to cure the problem because you still have the underlying adversarial role where one wants to theoretically prove as big an injury as possible, and the defense wants to prove as little an injury as possible.

I do believe that the adversarial nature of law, as it is involved in medicine, triples and quadruples the costs of medical treatment in care and examinations in those instances that involve litigation.

I think we need to educate people away from the litigation mentality that we all have, where "If a mistake is ever made concerning me, I deserve to get as much as I possibly can, no matter
what," and the question is, how do you do that? The law is there,
the opportunity is there, and people are going to say, "That person hurt me. They deserve to pay me something." Go down to
Mexico, for example, and walk around the streets and think in
terms of what that municipality faces as an exposure to litigation
based on the condition of the roads and the sidewalks. Then walk
around any big city in the United States, they're clean and don't
have the hazards of down there, and our cities and counties are
constantly being sued and collected against, for things like trip-
ping over a crack in the sidewalk. Somehow the people in Mexico
and the people in Europe survive without those lawsuits.

11

HMO MEANS "Hurry it up, Move 'em Out"

The trend seems evident—we are moving toward managed care, whether it is legislated or not. As more and more health-care consumers end up with this kind of coverage and the patient base drops for many independent physicians, doctors and other health-care practitioners are abandoning private practice and becoming employees of HMOs. While there seems to be universal tolerance of HMOs in theory, there is nearly universal dislike of the practice. The most-often expressed problem people have with this system is its rigidity, that every patient's symptoms must somehow conform to a list on a computer printout, and must somehow respond to treatment as recommended by that same printout. Yet, as everyone in the health-care field knows—there's no such thing as a textbook patient.

I keep hearing people say that the trend in health care is towards managed care. Whether we like it or not, it's going to happen.

Anytime you give anyone their money up front and then expect to get quality service back, I think you're deceiving yourself. To put it in an analogy, if you're going to add a room addition onto your house, do you pay the contractor every penny that he asks for before he puts the foundation in? If you do, I don't think you're going to see your room built. This is the same kind of thing that happens in HMOs.

These HMO clinics can really differ in quality. Some of them have x-ray equipment, some don't. Some have a well-trained, qualified staff, some maybe aren't so qualified. Even in patient care, some are concerned with the needs of the patient, some are just there to make money. Unless you work in health care, say you're the average patient, there's no way you'll know what you're getting.

HMOs—Health Maintenance Organizations. Socialized medicine for profit. An HMO operates on the capitation basis. They get "x" number of dollars per patient per year—period. They get all their money up front, and then it's a tug-of-war between the patient and the HMO over who gets the money. The more money they spend on your health care, the less money they get to keep.

The people who run HMOs, in many cases, are not health-care professionals, they're business people and insurance industry types. It's like a large corporation. You've got CEOs at the top and management personnel that have gone to school for business, not health care, and they're making decisions that impact on the health care of patients that they have no business making.

HMOs may have started out with the best of intentions. They may be honest and ethical, but at some point they are faced with a situation where if they provide the proper care, they're going to lose—for example, patients who are suspected of having cancer. With the proper tests and the cancer therapy, which could cost hundreds of thousands of dollars, they're going to lose money at the end of the year. So decisions are then made that are contrary to the patient's best interest. I have read firsthand accounts of physicians who have dropped out of HMOs for that very reason—

it became their job to keep the patient from receiving necessary health care.

The physician should never be in a situation where if he provides the quality of care required, he's penalized. What they have done is turned the physician from a patient's advocate to a patient's adversary. That's the reality of HMOs.

The only HMO with which I'm acquainted is the one with which I'm associated, [Kaiser] which is a group model rather than a staff model HMO.

There's a big philosophical difference there. Because I am not associated with a gatekeeper concept, and I'm not an HMO employee, being in the group model gives me the advantage of being in practice for myself in a setting where, while inevitably everyone is economically driven, I think there is less emphasis on the economics of the practice and more on excellence in practice.

We really don't have gatekeepers in our group. I would never function in that way. If somebody should be referred, I do it. If somebody insists on being referred even though they shouldn't be, I do. Those kind of problems occur more often in the staff model than the group model HMO.

As physicians, we don't work for the HMO. We don't work for the hospital or for the insurer. We work for us. We don't require permission to hospitalize. Obviously, if something is completely off the wall, it's going to be questioned, but generally we just admit. Our attitude is that the administration works for us. We do not work for them. In the staff model, it's the other way around. I have never been told that I could not admit a patient. Never been questioned in my life.

My one experience with the staff model HMO was with a patient that I ended up picking up who needed hospitalization. This patient had dual coverage, us and another HMO. I did what I always do, just put the patient in the hospital. No authorization was required for that at all. The patient's husband contacted the other health plan, and they got their approval nurse on the phone. To me, it was unbelievable the stuff that they asked. I just kept telling her, "Hey, look, this patient has Kaiser Health Plan, we're taking care of it."

But she wanted all the details to see if it would fit into a coverable illness. It was mindboggling compared to what we're used to.

The term "managed care" is misused in many instances. True managed care, my question would be, what is it? Does that take away the patient's right to manage their own care? Does it take away the family's right, or responsibility, to manage their own care? If we mean by managed care that we are looking at each individual that comes into the health-care system to see if their health care is managed appropriately, and we're looking at the history and the prognosis of that patient—what care is appropriate and ought to be given to that individual and is the best economical use of time, people and other resources—I'm all for it. Who wouldn't be for it? But it's very difficult to see that in what's called managed care.

I sit on some health care boards where I see "managed care" that is merely a quota system. For instance, how many home care visits can we allow? We should not allow more than six, or twelve, or fifteen, home care visits following "x" kind of a procedure. So here's a patient that really needs ten home visits but they're supposed to stop after six, and so just about regardless of what's going on, the visits are stopped at six.

I also know of instances where an individual should not be receiving home care, who's driving here and there but somehow can't get themselves into the physician's office or health-care clinic. There should be no way that person gets home care. Yet, under managed care systems built on quotas, they can get it.

All the physicians I've worked with have the same kinds of middle-of-the-night panics of "Did I make all the right decisions today?" That's one of the drawbacks in managed care. You end up having to see so many more people, you have less and less time to see the patient, so you have to make decisions quicker.

In the health maintenance organization type situation, attention is always placed on the areas that will affect the bottom line because at the end of the year those things determine the amount the physicians get in their profit-sharing plan. You know, reduce costs, keep that patient out of the hospital or get him out sooner, more is in that pot for you at the end of the year.

This HMO I do business with is really growing. The more they build, their profit sharing for the physicians goes up as well. They pay them a reasonable salary—it sounds low by California standards—and they give them specific objectives as far as cost containment. The doctors know where their bread is buttered. If they meet these goals every year, they have a big meeting out in the desert someplace, and the bonus that they pay these guys for meeting these objectives can easily amount to their full salary for the year. They can really end up making a good salary.

An HMO looks at patients differently than a private hospital would. Every time a patient is admitted to a private hospital, they look at that patient as income. Every time one is admitted to an HMO, they see that patient as a cost. The HMO has a vested interest in getting the best job done for the least amount of money.

The good part about managed care is that supposedly more people can get health care for less dollars, therefore the amount of dollars we're spending now goes further. The bad part of it is that the productivity is pushed and stretched to its maximum limits. You have your least qualified people doing more work than they're possibly qualified for.

What happens in the managed care situation is, the doctors get stretched very thin. They're seeing more patients and have less time to spend with each one. That leaves it up to the nurses, the technologists, the technicians, and to the greatest extent, their supporters, like runners—the people who transport patients from their rooms to radiology and back. You'll have fewer technologists because they're more expensive. Fewer nurses. You'll have more aide-type people, because they're paid less. So your least trained people will be doing the most for the patient. That's the problem with managed care.

The big concern now is how are we going to provide more health care to more people and still keep the overall financial picture at a reasonable level. I think that's real difficult. Every few weeks I receive an invitation to join another health plan as a preferred provider. Most of them are rather hideous. Their pitch is that they will provide more patients to me, they'll fill my office, but in turn they want me to slash my fees sometimes up to twenty-five percent. Some of them have considerable clout and sell a lot of plans to many employers, so you're in a bind sometimes, knowing that you'll see a drop in patient load if you do not accept the offer.

It forces you to involve more technicians in the examination process, go to shorter exam times, and see more patients per day to handle the increase in overhead. That's the way practices are moving right now. And it sounds like that's what Clinton's plan is going to force on all of us. If they cut my reimbursement fees across the board, I hate to say it, but I honestly don't think I can continue to provide the same quality of care that I do now.

There are some big clinics that will take every insurance no matter what the reimbursement is and run it like a mill, then the quality of care declines and people don't get what they need or want.

People come in and they have something in the back of their minds that they're worried about and that takes time to ferret it out. There's no time for reassurance, and so much of primary care is reassurance. "You're OK. Your health is OK." The more overcrowded a place gets the less you'll be able to do that for people. So then they'll keep coming back because they're still scared, and you won't ever have been able to get to the root of it because you still don't have the time or you don't ever see that person again, somebody else sees them.

W e had a lot of trouble because reimbursement was so low that we couldn't find specialists that would take certain PPO plans. We couldn't just look in the insurance book for a referral, we would have to call around. That takes our office staff time or our personal time, that takes money for us to do this. If I give the person a referral and then they find out that they're not on that plan, then that person comes back to the office and says to me, "Who else do you want to choose?" That all adds up.

W here has competition gone between hospitals? It's not from the technology side anymore, they don't advertise that any more because all of those departments have become cost centers rather than revenue centers. The fewer procedures they do, the better off they are.

Where the competition is now is for the managed care providers, the insurance companies. Is this hospital better for a particular HMO or PPO than that hospital? Do they have better surgeons? Do they have better equipment? Should I award my twenty thousand patients to this one, or shall I award them to that one because they have a full pediatric wing and a children's hospital? Those things help determine where a contract will be awarded, but the bottom line is, "Which hospital can make our plan the most profit?"

The insurance companies bargain on the money. How much will you do my twenty thousand patients for? They've gotten very crafty. They don't put all their eggs in one basket. They'll say, "Tell you what, we'll give your hospital seventy-five hundred patients, and we'll give this other hospital ten thousand, and we'll give another twenty-five hundred. And after a year, we'll renegotiate all this." Then what they'll do is see who manages those patient populations most efficiently—which translates into who they make the greatest profit off of—and then one may be out of the running, or another one may be out. That's where the competition is now.

T here is incredible frustration with insurance companies telling pharmacists that this patient cannot have this drug because he has this insurance plan. That's very common now. There's a list of drugs, called formularies, and the list is approved primarily with financial considerations in mind. Medicaid here in our state is a classic example of a closed formulary. If your physician chooses a drug that's very expensive, it's not covered, they will not pay for it. End of discussion. If you want it, you'll have to pay for it yourself. And it's not just government programs, private industry has adopted that methodology, HMOs are following the lead. They are limiting how well a patient can be treated.

Antibiotics are a very good example. I can use an old drug that sells for ten dollars or a new drug that's going to cost ninety. The ninety-dollar one kills more different kinds of bacteria than the ten-dollar one. Your case may be serious enough where you should have the ninety-dollar one, but if your insurance company, not knowing anything about you or your case, has already made the decision that all you can have is the ten-dollar prescription, you're going to suffer. There are going to be adverse effects.

Unfortunately, that's the trend. Therapeutic decisions are made on a financial basis, not a very good reason to decide. But yet, you only have so many dollars, the pie is only so big, it can only go so far.

One of problems that I see within ophthalmology happens to be cataract surgery. In the past, cataracts have been removed too early and because of that tendency, the government, Medicare, has put in guidelines where an individual cannot have them removed unless their vision is twenty/fifty or less. Twenty/ fifty is a fairly good size letter on the chart. Cataracts are really a subjective type of problem. For some patients—engineering types—twenty/forty would be hideous, but it may not bother another patient.

Now I'm noticing that HMOs are following the lead, and I've seen where an HMO will tell a patient to go home and come back next year when their vision is twenty/seventy or twenty/eighty. The cataracts could really be affecting the patient, but because of the HMOs budget constraints, the physician, under pressure of the HMO administration, will make the decision not to do the surgery at that point, not unless it's absolutely debilitating. It's just one less procedure and fewer dollars that the HMO has to expend at that time.

The way HMOs work, you pay a fee to belong to that organization and all your health care is covered, from an ingrown toenail to a brain tumor. But it's to their disadvantage to have a 500-bed hospital full of people all wanting or needing expensive tests. A patient says, "I have this recurring pounding headache and I'm having trouble seeing." The HMO answers, "Well let's see we can either get a skull series or an MRI. Tell you what, a skull series is a couple hundred bucks, an MRI is a thousand dollars." Are they going to want to do MRIs on everyone with that complaint? Hell no.

Just yesterday, a product rep was in here, she's a big opponent of HMOs. She saw this happen to a friend. Several years ago this friend had a cancerous growth on one of her hands. It had been cauterized off and treated with medication and had cleared up. Well it came back. She recognized it right away. It was a small skin cancer maybe the size of a quarter.

In the meantime, she had gone from private insurance to an HMO. When she goes to her HMO, the first thing she has to do is get past the gatekeeper, the physician in charge of seeing everyone first. If these gatekeepers let too many people up the ladder to specialists for too many exotic, or even necessary, tests, they get letters of reprimand.

So the gatekeeper said it didn't look like much to him. He gave her some kind of cream and sent her home. She called back right away because nothing happened and it was getting worse. Of course then she had to go through the whole thing again. She had to wait until the next opening which was another three or four weeks down the line.

Now the cancer was going a third of the way up her arm. The gatekeeper said, "Well, the cream didn't work." So he sent her to a dermatologist who said, "Try this cream." They wouldn't acknowledge that it might be cancer yet. They're still thinking it was some kind of psoriasis or ectopic dermatitis. Before this poor girl got to the cancer specialist, it had gone up her arm and was now going down her torso.

She's now on chemotherapy and may have to undergo radiation. All of this for a skin cancer that when it was first brought to their attention was smaller than the size of a quarter.

I know, I know, HMOs are wonderful because they look at the patient from a standpoint of prevention and health maintenance. That makes good sense, we probably can save substantial health-care dollars using that method. But my question is, how do you prevent accidents from happening? How do you prevent someone from slipping on the ice and breaking a rib and puncturing a lung and developing further complications? How do you stop genetic factors from playing into it? How do we prevent a woman with a history of breast cancer in her family from ever developing breast cancer? How about degenerative arthritis? Alzheimer's? Parkinson's? How do you prevent the aging process?

Preventive medicine and maintenance aren't going to solve every disease and injury, but HMOs are selling their worth on this idea that preventive medicine is the solution to all our health-care problems. In other words, if we could provide enough of preventive medicine, there would be no cost in health care beyond that. That's unrealistic. If you've got a system that's profitable only when you prevent illness from occurring and the majority of your clients are generally healthy, those who aren't healthy are going to find that the system fails them.

I'm going to sound rash in saying this, I suppose, but doesn't it seem logical that HMOs would want to get the unhealthy people out of the system as quickly as possible? If you can't benefit them by preventive care and maintenance, what are you going to do with them? You sure can't make a profit on them. The tendency then would be to help them die faster and save the system money.

From what I'm seeing and hearing—the horror stories that are becoming more and more common—I'm afraid that the gatekeeper is becoming the one forced to take the responsibility for deciding who to leave behind. If an HMO finds that their gate-keepers are dragging along too many patients that are a burden to the health of the organization, they have no qualms about letting those doctors go.

In a tribe of hunter/gatherers, it's justified by promoting the good of the whole group over the good of the individual. HMOs operate the same way. If they can prevent money being spent on the sick of their community, they can keep the costs down for the majority, and make a healthy profit for the owners and managers as well. Unfortunately, I wonder just how much of our illness and injury is preventable, in practical terms?

I worked in an HMO hospital as a nurse in the maternity ward. I remember one mother who had an extremely difficult time, just went through an extremely hard time with her delivery. It was hospital policy to discharge to home three hours after delivery. In many cases that's fine, but this woman was in no condition to go home. I protested to the doctor but he said she was capable of going home, that was the hospital policy, and he overruled my objections. They sent her home.

Several hours later she returned with massive hemorrhaging. She lost a lot of blood. She barely survived. That was the final straw for me. I quit. I just couldn't work for a hospital that cared more about costs than patient welfare any longer.

People who are used to a private doctor have been used to going where they want to go and if they're not happy they have the option of switching to somebody else. They figure it will be the same way at an HMO only everything will be cheaper. They expect the quality of the doctors is going to be the same. They get there and see you don't get a choice, you get funneled to whoever they want to give you to. And then the reason you're there is often ignored if it's going to be too great an expense to the system.

I have a friend who has a history of cancer. She's had bouts with it before. Four months ago she started having a lot of symptoms again, a lot of pain. She went to her HMO and they prescribed Motrin for her and kept telling her everything was fine, it was only arthritis. Apparently the pain from bone cancer and arthritis is quite similar.

She's finally been diagnosed with bone cancer and she started chemotherapy five days ago. She just got shoved around for four months. She was trying to tell them, but she couldn't get past the gatekeeper.

As a hospital, we're dealing more and more with health maintenance organizations. When a patient signs over their Medicare benefits, they no longer have co-pays and they no longer have deductibles and they no longer have the paperwork, but they also no longer have the right of choice. The health maintenance organization determines what hospitals they go to, what doctor they go to, how long they stay in the hospital and whether they'll have a particular benefit when they leave the hospital. We're finding more and more these resources are being limited, and we're going to be moving in that direction. That's part of the Clinton proposal, the use of health maintenance organizations.

I think it's the older folks who are getting raped the most by these senior HMO insurance plans. Many people don't have health insurance until they reach sixty-five and get on the Medicare system. And as soon as they do, these companies are coming to them and they get "Beth" to sign this and sign that, and now she has this plan and everything's OK. Well I'm sorry, but if Beth has an emergency and comes to our hospital instead of to their facility, and our call doesn't convince them that Beth needs to be seen here, she's out the door, to be seen maybe two or three days later.

Sometimes we get them on the phone and can really convince them by saying, "Listen, you're going to be held liable when this person has problems," but you're still fighting these authorization people.

You've got to understand, they're making a diagnosis over the phone without having seen the patient. Usually it's a nurse on the other end—it can be a physician. Some of these people work out of their homes. I know nurses who work out of their homes and are on-call for these authorization calls.

The liability for that patient falls on the hospital that the person walked into. That's the doctor who has seen them first. If that patient's insurance denies treatment and you let that person go and something happens to them, the insurance company isn't liable, the hospital is. Then, not only do you have to assume the expense of screening and treating the patient, you'll probably end up losing the lawsuit.

A re patients defrauded and purposely confused by commercial groups? Advertising is designed to get you to purchase a product, it's not designed to educate you. When you see these ads for HMOs they're designed to get you to walk into your doctor's office and sign over your Medicare check. If you notice, too, a lot of these commercials that have to do with health care, specifically HMOs for seniors, very few of them talk about what kind of care they provide. They talk about planting redwoods or something, and their pitch was, "No forms to fill out."

I talked with a woman seven or eight months ago, who told me, "I just came from visiting my mother. They talked my mother into joining one of those seniors' HMOs. They're going to kill my mother." She went through this whole story about when she took her mother into the HMO for a routine check. The doctor could hardly speak English. He gave her 500 pills to take that had nothing to do with her condition.

I said, "She can get her Medicare back. Tell her it takes thirty days. Tell her to drop out of this thing and go to the doctor and pay a little bit. You're going to get what you pay for, one way or the other." She said, "I tried that, but all of her friends in this retirement community are all under the same thing, and they all think it's great." Sure enough, I saw her again about three months later and she was close to tears. They had misdiagnosed her mother for months.

While she's telling me this, a gentleman overheard our conversation and he had to speak up. He said, "Yeah, a friend of mine just died from one of those seniors' HMOs. For two years they treated him for arthritis, and he had bone cancer. For two years they gave him Motrin. He had bone cancer, and they never detected it because they had never run the tests."

I hate to be cynical, but this is what is going on. If an HMO suspects bone cancer, or any other cancer, and does the tests to detect it, then they have to provide therapy and treatment. It's going to cost them a fortune. But if they can just give patients Motrin and stall them until they die, an HMO can make a profit. Would you want to have as your physician a man who would work under these circumstances, who would agree to these terms?

O ur neighbors have a daughter who was born with birth defects, spinal problems, cleft palate. She's been through specialists all these years and everything's been OK.

The dad works for the phone company, and his employer has now sent him to an HMO. The doctors are telling them that the girl doesn't need any more surgery. The HMO is also saying, "No, you can't see anymore specialists. We're not going to pay for it." So now, they're having to spend out of their own pocket what their insurance used to cover. They've had to go out and get loans just to see a doctor because their HMO will not look at her. This little girl has a file this thick, and they insist nothing is wrong with her.

W e just received a blanket statement issued by a seniors' HMO provider regarding the transfers of their patients from rural areas to hospitals. It says, "Regardless of patient condition, all transfers are to be routed through the local ground ambulance service."

This is ridiculous. From one area alone, the ground ambulance must make a treacherous hour and a half drive through mountainous terrain that is "radio silent" for the majority of the trip. Air transport from the same point to the hospital is fifteen minutes with full radio communications. Tell me that this doesn't constitute a real danger to such critical patients as trauma and heart attack victims. But the HMO, in order to control costs, has made this policy that not only fails to take into consideration the specific needs of an individual, it actually threatens lives.

We had an HMO subscriber transferred from his local ER to our hospital via helicopter after being diagnosed with an acute myocardial infarction and having thrombolytic therapy initiated. Following his successful treatment and subsequent release, he was informed by the HMO's representative that the air transport in his case was deemed "unnecessary" and would not be covered. The HMO determined, in all their wisdom, that because his wife was present with him, she could have driven the two and a half hours between his ER and our hospital for his cardiac care. Come on! The standard of care for all acute MI patients is to have an IV, oxygen administered, cardiac monitoring, and trained medical personnel in attendance whenever you transfer. Simply put, the two and a half hour drive in the family car for this patient represents a death sentence mandated by that HMO.

A friend of mine, another nurse, who works at another hospital in town, told me this story just this evening. About four days ago, a 72-year-old woman presented herself to her HMO office with a chief complaint of chest pain. She was seen briefly by the physician and then sent home after an EKG was done and lab specimens were drawn. The doctor, who was not a cardiologist, probably interpreted her EKG as within normal limits. He didn't see the obvious signs of a heart attack taking place and rather than admit her for observation, he sent her home. Here's an example of a gatekeeper's inadequate evaluation turning away someone who needed treatment for a serious complaint. This is quite common in HMOs.

Later that same day, someone from the HMO office called this patient at home and directed her to go to the nearest emergency room "right away." She was told that something had "showed up" on her lab results and she needed to be checked further. What that something was elevated cardiac enzymes which is indicative of a heart attack. So the doctor made a mistake. But rather than direct her to call 911, she was instructed to drive to the nearest emergency room. She should have been transported by ambulance. Why would you instruct a patient who is having a heart attack to drive to the nearest emergency room rather than call for an ambulance? Could it be to save costs?

Upon her presentation to a local emergency room, she was diagnosed with an acute inferior wall myocardial infarction which is a very serious heart attack. The patient was then admitted to the Intensive Care Unit for observation.

Three days later, the patient was discharged home. Just three days later. The standard of care is to observe known heart attack patients for at least five days because the dying cardiac tissue involved in the heart attack begins to decompose and break down after three to five days, causing further life-threatening problems. But early discharge of critical HMO patients is a common practice. The HMO will only pay so much, regardless of the individual patient's condition and if the hospital is not going to be reimbursed, they'll end up complying and discharging the patient before they should.

This morning, the day after her premature discharge from the hospital, the patient returned to the same emergency room via paramedic ambulance. At this point, she was in severe cardiogenic shock. Despite all the vigorous attempts to stabilize this patient, she is not expected to survive. The patient's current grave condition will prevent any restorative measures which may have been implemented if the patient had been properly monitored in the hospital throughout the "critical time" following her heart attack.

This patient will probably die needlessly. All her managed care plan really accomplished was that it "managed" to kill her in spite of what proper medical treatment could have provided.

For an HMO, every time a patient comes in it loses money. They make more money by not seeing patients. Supposedly when the HMO system came in, it was intended to keep people healthy. You know, come in for your routine checks. But even then, they actually lose money. They really lose money when one of their patients goes to an emergency room that's not listed in their plan. Then they have to take money out of their pocket and pass it on to the other hospital. They'll do anything to prevent that from happening.

Let's say Medicare is paying them $500 to take care of Mr. Jones. But if Mr. Jones comes to an emergency room and it costs $1,000, they've actually lost $500, so they discourage these treatments. This causes their negative responses of "We won't authorize payment for treatment. Where we really want to treat that patient is . . . ," or, "Are you sure that it's absolutely necessary?" If a patient needs help, they want them to come only to their facilities because those costs are already included in their overhead. It doesn't cost them the extra money.

I 'm a registered nurse. I've been doing it for seven years, the last year and a half in the emergency room. I think the health-care system we have now is good, most people coming into the hospital are getting the treatment they need. It's the insurance companies that seem to be the problem. You know, people coming in who really need treatment, yet they can't be treated because they're on an HMO. Either, they've got to be shipped out, or it's "not something we can authorize the patient to be seen for."

It's done to prevent people from coming into an emergency room because they've got a runny nose or a cough. I can understand that. But the guidelines have gotten so strict that you basically have to sell the insurance provider a picture of how sick this person is before they'll allow you to treat the patient. And this causes problems.

Hospitals are required to abide by COBRA [commonly known as the "antidumping" law]. That means when anyone comes in, no one can be refused treatment, regardless of the hospital's ability to collect payment from the individual. However, if you want to get paid, HMOs have to give authorization before you can treat. But because of COBRA laws, when a person comes into a hospital, they have a right to be treated. As a result, hospitals are incurring costs that they may never be reimbursed for. The hospital's emergency room physician is going to see the patient, the nursing staff is going to triage the patient. There's clerical time, time on

the phone to the insurance company, supplies—extensive expense
to the hospital as soon as that patient walks through the door.

The patient is brought through the system and no money is
given to the hospital for doing the screening, unless it's a severe
problem. The only HMO now that does allow screening is Kaiser—at least the hospital gets something. Kaiser's the only company that a patient can come into our private hospital, we'll screen
them, and then they will talk, ER doctor to ER doctor, and say,
OK, we'll send a transfer team, or send the patient over to the
Kaiser hospital, or whatever. And it behooves them. If a person's
got asthma, then let's quickly evaluate them, give them one treatment, and then send them over to Kaiser for the rest of their treatment. It's not an all or nothing thing where they're either totally
seen here or not seen at all. Unfortunately, that's generally the
case with all other HMOs.

I'd say, of the insurance patients who come in, fifty percent or
more are patients who are on an HMO that need authorization
before you can do anything. Our hospital guidelines are, we triage
them to see what their problems are. Do they need to be brought
in right away? Then we register them. Then even if they get denied we have a physician who comes over and looks at them first.
Because we did have a case where a woman was denied authorization, we looked at her real quick and sent her out the door. She
had an aneurysm and died.

Who got sued? Us, the hospital. Not the authorizing doctor or
nurse who said, "No, you can't treat her there. It just sounds like
a migraine. She was already seen yesterday. Give her some more
Tylenol and send her home."

Sometimes we have to threaten to put an HMO authorization
person into the emergency room to get them to authorize
treatment. You know, "If you don't OK this, I'm going to hunt
you down and break every bone in your body."

A thirteen-year-old girl was brought into our ER by private
auto a few weeks ago. She had been accidentally hit on the side
of the head with a golf club during gym class. At the time she was

conscious and demonstrated no adverse symptoms. Even though she was asymptomatic, you have to be very careful with injuries to the head. Some serious conditions might not show up for a day or two, and by the time they do, it could be too late.

But before we could run any diagnostic tests, we had to obtain payment authorization from her HMO. They refused. They said, "She doesn't have any symptoms. Send her home." Our ER doc had to get on the phone and scream at them that the possibility of a skull fracture did exist and that he felt it absolutely necessary to check. The impact of a golf club to the head was sufficient to cause a fracture and the only way to rule it out was to x-ray it.

They still denied authorization. Whatever they had on their little list in front of them said, unless the patient has this and this and this, we will not pay for it. It was only because of our ER doc's badgering and threatening, that they finally acceded to his demands.

A skull x-ray was performed and the results showed a depressed skull fracture. Such an injury requires at least a 24 hour hospitalization for observation, and this has to be in a facility with neurological capability. Our hospital didn't have a neurosurgeon on staff so we urged that the patient be transferred to a facility that did. The HMO refused to authorize the patient's transfer to the closest available facility which was fifty miles away. They directed us to discharge the patient and send her home.

Our ER doctor went through the roof. I've never seen him so mad. After two hours of bitter telephone conversations—two hours, during which he was on hold a good deal of the time—the HMO finally agreed to authorize the girl's transfer. As it turned out, within 24 hours her condition deteriorated to the point that emergency neurosurgery had to be performed.

The only reason that patient is probably alive today is because our ER doctor refused to take no for an answer. If that HMO's instructions had been followed, that girl would probably have died at home, or at least suffered permanent disability. And in either of those cases, you can bet that it would have been our hospital and staff that would have been sued for malpractice. Not the HMO.

O h, we had a horrible case the other night. A young guy, thirty-two years old, was brought into the ER by ambulance. It was a motorcycle accident, and judging by the way he looked, he must of skid a couple miles down the highway after his bike went down. He was a mess. Didn't have a helmet on.

When he was initially triaged, we noted that he was unresponsive and his pupils were dilated and fixed. But he was still breathing on his own and his cardiac rhythm was normal.

He was under an HMO, which meant that after our initial screening and stabilizing of the patient, we had to call and get authorization for payment of services. The HMO refused. The representative said that it was not an emergency and would not authorize payment for services. I guess she thought that it would be foolish to spend any money on a patient who was going to die anyway.

I t just makes me wonder, seeing what we go through in our ER to treat HMO patients, how many of them suffer or are put in a life-threatening situation because somebody removed from the situation makes a decision regarding their treatment over the phone based on insurance guidelines rather than the patient's condition. It's a foolish, impractical, and dangerous way to practice medicine.

I don't want the quality of care for myself or my family that I've seen HMOs provide routinely. I won't tolerate it. If I have to go to a black market to get decent health care, I'll do that. Under Clinton's plan with its further push toward managed care, who knows, you may see a black market in medical care spring up.

I t's possible though, that some of the problems with HMOs will be addressed. Recently Health Net [California's second-largest HMO] was ordered to pay damages to the family of a breast cancer patient who died after being denied treatment—in this case a bone marrow transplant, which was covered by her policy. Health Net said this treatment for breast cancer was experimental, but the jury apparently felt this was based solely on saving the company money. Well, the jury awarded the victim's family a total of $99.1 million! And when the judge announced the award he said the case was clear-cut and that corporations can't claim to provide a benefit and then try to get out of providing it. This was a really big breakthrough for consumers because it puts these companies on notice that they can't rake in your premiums and then deny you coverage you've already paid for.

12

THE EUTHANASIA OF THE INDEPENDENT PHARMACY

The corner drugstore may be a symbol of a bygone era but, as the speakers point out, they remain an essential part of the health-care system; often they are the last safeguard from errors before a patient actually commences treatment. With the growing emphasis on cost containment, big business interests are quickly squeezing out the smaller independent concerns that offer not just a product, but an invaluable service as well. Certainly this trend is not limited to pharmacies—the independent medical-equipment-and-supply companies are caught in the same bind— but they were the best example of what many of small health-care providers are facing.

The big money interests, and I include government in that, are putting us out of business. It's getting to be more difficult every day to keep the doors open. Independent health-care providers are being killed off. Government and big business claim we're dying anyway, so they're just doing us a favor by speeding up the process. Well, I can tell you, I know that when the small, independent health-care provider is gone, we're going to lose the last vestige of humanity in our health-care system.

R emaining totally honest is getting really tough. The only way
I can survive in health care is if I have accounts that want to
support me because they feel I do good work and offer the best
service for their patient. If you can find providers like that who
aren't only concerned about profit for themselves, there's a
chance of survival. It's getting harder and harder to compete
against the mega companies. I don't know how long it will be
before I can't.

I 'm a community pharmacist. When a patient comes in with a
prescription, the first thing we do is ascertain that this is the
proper dosage and so forth for the patient. We have to then check
against the previous record—we keep complete detailed records
of all prescriptions for drug interactions, contraindications, and
other potential problems that might come up. Then of course, we
select the proper product, dispense it and counsel the patient in
proper usage, storage, what to expect, what side effects might occur. My closing sentence is always, "If you have any problems,
call me."

The comments I get from a lot of patients is that this is something you don't see much any more, which I think is a shame. In
the chain or HMO level, you're treated so much like a number,
but in a community pharmacy, you're treated like a patient, which
is what you really are.

P harmacists aren't selling a product; what the pharmacist sells
is a service, a knowledge base. The physician writes a prescription, hands it to the patient, the patient takes it down to the
pharmacy. The pharmacist makes a separate evaluation as to the
appropriateness of that prescription.

It's easier when the pharmacist knows the patient because he
knows about them, what medical conditions they've had. He
knows more about what's happening to them now if he has a
personal relationship with that patient. But even if they're total
strangers, he knows a given number of things. If the patient is an
adult, for example, compared to a child, he evaluates whether the

dose and the drug are appropriate. If you have a 250-pound person should they get a different dose than a 35-pound baby? Well,
yeah, they probably should.

Is this a one-time-a-day pill or is this a four-times-a-day pill?
The pharmacist knows what it's supposed to be, what it usually
is. He compares what this document says, the prescription, with
what his database of knowledge is. The pharmacist makes all of
those evaluations and the patient never knows about it. A pharmacist spends, depending on where you are, minimum of five
years and oftentimes six or seven years preparing for what he
does.

P harmacists are a safeguard. It's not our job to diagnose and
second-guess the physician, it is our job to make sure that
the physician orders the proper drug. Even though the physician
goes to school for eight or nine years, studying drugs is really a
very small part of that education. However, when he's practicing
medicine, he ends up spending most of his day writing prescriptions. Doctors are human like everybody else and they can make
mistakes. That's part of the pharmacist's job, to safeguard the
patient against those mistakes, like prescribing the wrong drug
or dosage.

T he thing about pharmacists being a safeguard—it's really
true. And there's nothing that can substitute for face-to-face
contact with someone who knows you and your history.

Now all these mail-order pharmacies have 800-numbers and
pharmacists to call with questions, but the initiative has to come
from the patient, and often that's a problem. Patients put their
trust in us, and don't often feel they're in a position to question.
Too, they might not know they should ask if they feel something's
different. The other problem is things like potential drug interactions. For example, most mail-order drugs are long-term; you're
more likely to get the antibiotic you need locally. If you don't keep
everyone informed, you could have a situation where there's a
potentially dangerous drug interaction that neither the mail-order
pharmacist or the local pharmacist could know about.

I n the public opinion polls that ask what profession do you trust the most, pharmacy has come in number one in terms of honesty and the highest ethics the last five years in a row. We earned that. We play a vital role in the community: face-to-face.

Pharmacists have come in number one because they're accessible and they're free. If you ask your doctor a question, he's going to charge you an office visit for it, where the pharmacist and his knowledge is available to you by dialing the telephone.

The public still has tremendous trust in the people who give them drugs. They have to. You have to have some confidence that the pill you're going to take is what it says it is and that it's going to do what it's supposed to do. Everywhere along the line, the people have earned the consumer's trust—the manufacturer, the distributors, the pharmacist, the doctor who wrote it. There has to be trust or the whole system breaks down.

I worked for about seven years, saving my nickels and dimes, to open my own store—the American dream. In 1983 we took the big chance and opened our own store in a small community in the mountains of southern California. From the very beginning, it's been lots of hard work, being here for the patients, coming down after hours when there's emergencies. I've been here at three o'clock on a Sunday morning for emergencies. These are the things that we did to help the business grow.

We're now in our eleventh year. We have had tremendous response from the community. The other pharmacy in town had closed in November of 1982 and we couldn't get open until May of '83, so they went through one entire winter with no pharmacy here in this small town. We get a lot of snow up here sometimes, a lot of fog. It's difficult to have to drive down the hill, especially if you're sick, to get a prescription filled, so they were happy to have a pharmacy back.

For the first three years everything went well, then we started having trouble, and the trouble came from the insurance companies. It's a little-known fact, but in 1945 the McCarran/Ferguson Act exempted the insurance companies from the antitrust laws. These insurance companies, this $2 trillion industry, is protected from people like myself by this exemption. They can engage in practices that if I got together with other pharmacists and did, I'd end up in prison. They can collude. They can fix prices. They can divvy up markets. They're doing all of that.

In any given free market system, you're going to have those that are heavier into service and quality of product, and those that cut corners and put out a cheap product at a lower price. The public can choose which they want and anything in between. That's as it should be.

In pharmacy, what started to happen is those of us that were providing a higher quality of level of service, which of course costs more—coming down after hours, deliveries, going the extra distance to provide the level of service that people really want—we're going to be penalized now, because the insurance companies have figured that, since they contract for hundreds of thousands of people at a time, they're only going to pay the discount price. The deep discount, no frills, no service, that's it, kind of concept. Well, if you're providing a level of service that can't survive on this kind of price or reimbursement, you can't accept these insurance plans.

We're talking about all the major insurance intermediaries. They started discounting. First they used to pay what was called the wholesale price, plus a certain fee—say the wholesale price plus four dollars. Well, they started to discount the wholesale price. First they took off five percent, then they took off ten, and then twelve. I've seen contracts as low as the wholesale price minus eighteen percent plus maybe two dollars. What that means is that a pharmacist who's responsible for the well-being of the patients that come in here—to check for drug interactions, who had to go through years of school, who is legally liable should something go wrong—he's going to get paid less to fill a prescription than the average hardware store owner gets for selling a hammer. Now there's something wrong with that kind of system. If you sign these contracts that turn over control of your pricing structure to a third party, especially a third party as callous as the insurance industry, don't be surprised that as time goes by they keep lowering what they're going to pay you. Once you're dependent upon them, they own you. You're going to be nothing more than an indentured servant to the insurance industry. That's where we're at today.

The insurance companies are calling the shots, setting the fees and always pricing at rock bottom. That's why in the last eighteen months in California alone, eighteen percent of the independent pharmacies have closed their doors. This does not bode well, especially for small communities that rely on pharmacists. I know in our community I'm the first health professional a lot of folks are going to see. In many cases, I'm the only one they'll see. They can't afford to see a doctor, or they don't want to bother. Or, what I'm seeing more and more of, they're in an HMO, they can't be seen for three, four, or five weeks. If the man in the trenches, the independent pharmacist who's out there in the small communities, if he's lost, then a lot of small communities are going to lose a very valuable asset.

As an independent community pharmacist, I am finding it impossible to compete with the mail-order houses. There are two main reasons for this: multi-tier pricing and price-fixing by the insurance companies.

The independent community pharmacies are on the verge of extinction. We can't compete against the advantages that HMOs and mail-order pharmaceutical companies are given, given by the government by the way—and they're supposed to be the champions of the small businessman? The government is practicing euthanasia on a lot of unwilling victims. If you kill the independent health-care provider, our whole health-care system is going to die.

In the marketplace there's the concept that if you have a chain of drug stores, these drug stores can buy huge volumes of medicines and therefore they're entitled to a discount for buying a large volume. No complaints with that. If a manufacturer can sell to one man who's going to buy a million pills as compared to a thousand people who, combined, would only buy a million pills, it's going to cost the manufacturer less to sell it to the big account. That makes perfectly good sense to me and I take no offense at that whatsoever.

But what we have in pharmacy is called multi-tier pricing. I'll use product names because there are a couple of really good examples. One is Coumadin. It's a blood thinner. It's critical to the people who need it. When I, an independent pharmacist, buy Coumadin at wholesale, it costs about $44 for a hundred pills. But, if I work for a not-for-profit hospital that's right across the parking lot, I can buy it for 44 cents. If you can manufacture that product and sell it to the hospital for 44 cents and you're selling it to me for $44, there's something wrong. The hospital does not buy a thousand times as much as I do. There's simply a limited number of patients who need this particular drug. So there has to be some other reason why you're selling at two markedly different prices. And there is. You, the drug manufacturer, want to make sure that all the physicians get trained to use your brand name drug.

It's like Tylenol in the hospital. When I worked at County, we would buy it in barrels, literally in barrels. We would scoop it out with a flour scoop. They were so cheap that there was no reason to ever count them and we would literally dispense them in gallon jars, they were that cheap for us. The manufacturer was selling it at so little to train everyone to use Tylenol rather than acetaminophen. They wanted that Tylenol name to stick. They were giving financial incentives to institutions to train everyone there that Tylenol was the brand, and it's worked very, very well. On commercial advertisements, they claim to be the most prescribed drug. But there's a reason—it's so cheap you can't afford not to use it.

It's a good product, it's not that at all. It's that there are financial incentives to institutions to reward them for using some given brand, and they are unfair incentives. I have to compete at $44 with somebody who's buying it for 44 cents? I can't compete there. It's not a matter of volume. If I buy and sell as many as the hospital does, I still cannot get it at the price they get it at.

Pharmacists lost a big lawsuit that set pharmacy back by more than a decade. It's been thirteen years now since that lawsuit, and it was only this summer that similar new lawsuits were refiled in both state and federal courts. But once a federal court rules against you, it's over. The Supreme Court is the only other step. You run out of money and you simply cannot keep fighting.

If the courts rule that it meets a social good to have this multiple pricing system, the war's over. You've lost. It's OK to sell to this fellow at one-hundredth of what you sell it to the next fellow. Both are held to the same standards and quality of care. The price is the only difference and it's simply not a fair system. Congress is now giving consideration to this. The last couple of sessions have been lobbied heavily by pharmacy groups. If someone buys ten million pills a year and I only buy a thousand a year, they deserve a better price, but they don't deserve a price that's a hundred times better than mine. Whatever the playing field is going to be, just make it the same for everybody. Make everybody play by the same rules, whatever the rules may be, just make them the same for everyone.

S ometimes these multi-tier prices can be a difference of ninety percent. I have lists that date back years ago of the prices that are charged to me and what's charged to an HMO or to mail-order pharmacy.

A fellow, let's just call him Mr. Jones, came in to tell me that he stopped buying from me because he could get his nitroglycerin patches through the mail at a substantial savings. So I asked him to bring down the invoice, and he did. He was charged $24 for a box of thirty nitroglycerin patches. My cost at the time was almost $38, so I was charging him $44. I'm making six bucks and I'm $20 higher than what he was paying through the mail.

I have a couple of HMO pharmacists that work for me relief, they say that sometimes they pay a penny a patch. I pay a dollar a patch. They're paying $4 for the box of thirty, they sell it for $24, they've made a $20 profit. Is it right that they make a 500- or 600-percent profit, and I'm the bad guy because I'm charging $44 and I'm making six? I'm making a profit of about what? Twelve percent? Thirteen percent? That's not enough to keep this business going, but I'm perceived as price gouging. And yet it's over something that I have no control.

The National Association of Retail Druggists has been fighting for years to get this discriminatory pricing stopped. If a manufacturer can sell their patches to a mail-order house for $4 a box and make a profit, why do they have to charge me $36?

This is how I think it came about. You had the founder and CEO of Medco Cost Containment Services. My hunch is that he said, "Look, I've got this mail-order house we're going to start up. We're talking about ten thousand scripts a day here down the road, and I don't want to pay this price that everybody else is paying. I want a little break."

OK, so they gave him a little break. That's a small start, a little stream of discounts going to one company. Pretty soon, you've got mail-order houses popping up everywhere, and they all want the same price break. What was one or two percent of a manufacturer's business is now becoming ten or fifteen—my guess now is that it might be as high as twenty-five or thirty percent. The HMOs and the hospitals want the same deal as the mail-order house. Everyone is getting a break except the community retail pharmacy, be it chain or independent. We're stuck paying outrageous prices while everyone else involved in health care that deals with pharmaceuticals is getting a phenomenal discount.

I filled a prescription for a woman, 250 milligrams per five cc, 150 cc, a ten-day supply. She paid me, she went home, she submitted the claim to the workers comp.

Rather than sending the check to the patient, they sent it to me, the pharmacy. Under law, if the patient pays for the medication up front and submits a claim, they have to pay the patient what the pharmacy charged. However, if the pharmacy submits the claim, then the insurance provider is free to determine what the price should be. In other words, the bureaucrats determine what the fair price is for this. By sending me the check, which they shouldn't have done, they went through their normal process and fixed the price at what they thought was appropriate.

As you can see my price was $53.30. Well, they subtracted $17.31 saying that I had overcharged and sent me a check for $35.99. It says right here, "We have paid the attached bill in accordance with the division of Workers' Compensation official medical fee schedule and/or the medical legal fee schedule recommended by administrative director and [company's name] policies and guidelines." There's note number two. On the back it says, "The charge exceeds an amount that would appear reasonable." In other words some bureaucrat, the administrative director of their policies and guidelines has determined that my price was unreasonable.

Here is the invoice for what I have paid for that medication. The suggested wholesale price is $49.69. My actual acquisition cost after all my discounts was $43.27. They paid me $35.99. They paid me roughly $8 less than I actually paid for that myself. So I presume I'm expected to select the proper drug, get it ready, counsel the patient, check for drug interactions, contraindications and so forth, and kick in eight bucks. This is why more and more pharmacists are dropping out of these kind of insurance programs.

Now is somebody somewhere getting this same drug for $20 a bottle? I don't know. I don't have access to that kind of data. But if some bureaucrat someplace thinks this is a fair price, he must have some reason. The only reason I can think of is that somebody someplace is getting this at a marked discount, such that $35.99 will provide them with a decent profit.

I f things continue to go in the direction they seem to be heading and I'm limited to making fifty cents on a prescription while insurance companies and mail-order houses make millions in profits, I may just turn this place into a health food store.

M ail-order pharmacies have one purpose—it's making money. They don't want to deal with the patient, they just want to sell the product and make a profit, that's why they work through the mail. They put as much distance between themselves and the patient as possible. They're not a health-care provider, they're a supply house.

The Health Care Financing Administration commissioned a study done by people at Brandeis and Tufts that looked at the cost savings that mail-order pharmacies had to offer. When all the dust settled and the other costs were looked at, there weren't any. It cost every bit as much as the other systems where the patient had direct interaction with the pharmacists.

Do you know what the total compensation in 1992 was for the owner and CEO of the largest mail-order pharmaceutical house? Thirty point two million dollars. He's the seventh-highest paid CEO in the nation. Now in a country where we supposedly have 34 million people without health insurance, you're funneling over $30 million to one person? This is insane.

I'll give them some benefit of the doubt. I think this is what might have happened. Say, hypothetically, you make a calcium channel blocker. These are brand new, they're used for high blood pressure, and they don't have many side effects. There are several companies that have one or two out, and there's no generics yet, so they're all single-source drugs.

Now how do you get your product in volume into say hospitals, HMOs, or mail-order houses? You have to give a discount. The maker of one calcium channel blocker will try to undercut his competitor. So if they're going to sell it for twenty bucks a hundred, and that accounts for twenty percent of their sales, they've got to jack up the other eighty percent of sales by ten percent. That's how the prices really got out of control. I think once it got started, they just couldn't stop it. They can't stop it themselves, because if they were to stop, then in their minds their competitors would just take over that share of the market.

The companies that get these big discounts play one drug manufacturer against another. I saw a story in the *Wall Street Journal* about the deal that Medco got going with SmithKline Beecham to push its ulcer drug Tagamet over Zantac, the one made by Glaxo. What happens is, in exchange for the discount,

Medco puts the drug on its "Prescriber's Choice" list, which means that every time they receive a prescription for Zantac in the mail, they call the physician and lobby him into changing it. Now you see where this is going? The patient at this point is totally irrelevant to these people. They have banks of pharmacists who call physicians and try to convince them to change the prescription, that's all they do.

This Prescriber's Choice list actually started with the ulcer drug and now has something like eight drugs on it. What's interesting is that these are all brand-name switches. They're all under patent which means that chemically equivalent generics aren't available. So if you get switched, while the new drug would be similar, it wouldn't be the same. That means your doctor has to be pretty savvy about the chemical makeup of the different drugs, because while a switch may be fine for one patient, it may not be for another. And remember, too, when these people call the doctor, they don't really know much about you. Their point is, they're getting a discount on one manufacturer's brand but not on another, so every time they get that other manufacturer's script for that product, they'll call and try and talk the physician into changing it.

O ur state has laws regarding the use of technicians and ancillary personnel and interns in a pharmacy. One to one. One pharmacist to one tech. Other states have various laws, some have fewer restrictions than others. So while you may think, "Well, my state has strict laws and will check up on things," well, think again, because they don't necessarily apply. Some states make mail-order houses abide by their own laws, others don't. So all the laws that we have to abide by, that are designed to protect the consumer, as soon as you go across the state line to buy medications through the mail, all those laws and regulations may not apply.

If you're buying medications from out-of-state, you're buying from people you'll never know. You're willing to buy drugs that can put you in the hospital or worse from someone three thousand miles away? This doesn't make sense to me.

P harmacists are required by law in our state to offer mandatory patient consultation. This isn't something we choose; we
have to do it. But if a mail-order pharmaceutical house is located
out-of-state, they may be in a state where they don't have to counsel. How in the hell can I be held to a higher standard of care
when they're not? I am not objecting to the standard of care to
which I'm held. I'm simply stating that every single pharmacist
who dispenses to that patient should be held at the same level.

L ate in 1987 a lady out in Idaho ordered a prescription
through the mail. Her husband's employer had enrolled
them in a health-care plan where they could get their drugs
through the mail.

She bought the one prescription through the mail, it was supposed to be Prednisone. When she died of a cerebral hemorrhage
several months later, a blood-thinning drug called Coumadin was
found in her bloodstream in toxic levels. Coumadin is an antico-
agulant. The most common use other than in medicinal purposes
for patients who have trouble with phlebitis or blood clots is as a
rat poison. It causes them to bleed internally and die. The woman
had never had Coumadin prescribed for her, and she had never
ordered it.

The prosecutor in her area, Latah County, brought a felony
charge of involuntary manslaughter against the company. So here
you had this little county suing National Rx Services (part of
Medco) this huge mail-order house with a plant in Nevada. According to the prosecutor, on the first court date a stretch Mercedes pulled up in front of the courthouse and four pinstriped
attorneys got out. They then filed so many motions that he would
have used his whole budget for the year just answering these, so
he had to drop the case. All along Medco had denied any wrongdoing, claiming that the mixup may have occurred after the bottle
had left the plant. And the Nevada department of investigation
found no evidence of wrongdoing on the part of Medco. But I
have a hard time understanding how Coumadin got into a Prednisone bottle unless somebody at National Rx made a big mistake. Interestingly, the papers reported that Medco gave the

county $5,000 to help defray the costs of the suit and took steps
to revamp its dispensing system.

In the late eighties, there was a Senate subcommittee hearing
on mail-order pharmacies. Three pharmacists who had all
worked at one company testified from behind a screen. They said
they had quit in frustration over the "suicidal" pace at which they
were expected to sign off on prescriptions—fifty an hour acccord-
ing to one—mistakes they had caught in the dispensing of pills
and fears about mistakes maybe they hadn't caught. At the same
hearing a woman testified about sending for medicine for her hy-
pertension and getting a blood thinner instead, which could have
killed her. While a lot of noise was made about this at the time,
unfortunately, the hearings never went anywhere.

I had a woman once come in, a very dear friend of mine, a
teacher at the local school district, a school district with a plan
that uses mail-order. She came in with a letter she'd got one day
from her mail-order pharmacy and it asked her to describe the
tablets she had received, their color, size and shape. Apparently
they had sent her the wrong stuff and didn't know what they had
sent her and were trying to find out without letting her know what
had happened.

She said, "Could this be why I've been having so much trouble with my heart lately? My doctor can't figure this out." So not
only was she not taking what she was supposed to be taking for
the heart, but who knows, what she was taking might have adversely affected her heart. There's no way to tell because she had
already taken the whole bottle and gotten a refill.

How do pharmaceutical manufacturers get even with mail-
order houses? You've probably been reading about it in
the papers. They're merging with them. They're taking over the
whole thing.

Merck is merging with Medco Containment Services (the
irony is that until recently Merck was one of the loudest critics of

Medco's discounting schemes) and thrown in with this deal happens to be one of the large third-party administrators, which
Medco bought in 1985. So the largest pharmaceutical manufacturer picked up the largest mail-order house in the country along
with this third-party processing firm. Those are things that should
be kept distinctly different. Manufacturers should not be owning
pharmacies any more than doctors should.

So, if you are a pharmacist that buys from that wholesaler,
and you fill a prescription for a patient handled by this third-
party intermediary, you in essence will have the same company
determining the price you pay and the price you receive. How can
this happen? In a country where Ma Bell was supposed to break
up because they monopolized an industry, how you can allow the
largest manufacturer in the world to merge with the largest pharmacy in the world? I don't understand it. It doesn't make sense.

The antitrust watchdog seems to still be asleep. The change
of presidents didn't make any difference. There has been HR9
and Senate 430 before Congress for four years. These bills address the antitrust exemption, trying to revoke it, but nothing is
happening because, guess what, the insurance companies have a
lot more money than health-care providers.

13

IS GOVERNMENT QUALIFIED TO DIAGNOSE AND TREAT?

In asking this question the answer we most often heard was a resounding, "No." This answer is based on two incontrovertible pieces of evidence—the experiences that people have had dealing with HMOs and the government's track record in administrating large, bureaucratic programs. However, there seems to be universal acceptance of the fact that change of some sort will occur and an equally universal inability to prescribe an alternative to the Clinton proposal. Most health-care workers are adopting a wait-and-see attitude, while fearing the worst.

The biggest caution is, watch out for the superficial evidence. The media do not delve into something. They get soundbites and these become the answer. This is too complex. If anything, don't panic, don't try to solve the whole problem now.

Clinton started off with the right kind of concepts regarding managed competition, but the basic problem with the Clinton proposal is that it is typical of what we do in America. We identify the crisis, and then we need to have instant gratification. And so he's got to have a bill in 1994, and certainly by 1996 because of the election. That drives the whole thing. So, regardless of certain other considerations, we've got to do this.

In my opinion, if you really sit back you'll see that this is an evolutionary process. Why don't we examine where we want to be at a given point, what we identify as an ideal way to deliver health care from what we know right now, and where we want to go. What are the barriers to getting there? Where do we have laws and regulations and mismatched incentives that prevent us from having that type of care? Then eliminate those.

You can do that over a period of time, and you can test your theories. A big issue with the Clinton proposal is that it's ninety percent untested theories. It was said at one of our meetings, if the Clinton proposal is four percent in error on its funding, that will be a $5 billion cost to the country by 1998. That's only four percent. The estimate of the cost of Medicare was 700 percent off what they predicted when that came in, in 1966. So you've got to figure that there's going to be a huge error. Unfortunately with the election process, Clinton is not going to be the one held responsible at that time.

One other factor is that the country now is far less able to absorb a $5 billion error than we were in 1966 when the economy was on the "every year we're richer and better" trend. I think Congress is going to be more cautious this time around than they were when Medicare was legislated.

I think the best thing that Clinton has going for him is the fact that he has no rules yet. He's just watching everybody clamor around and hoping something will fall out. I don't think anyone knows what they really want to do. They just know that we need reform, so now there's fifty different types of reform going on and he'll take credit if it works and distance himself if it doesn't.

It's all coming about at a good time. Everybody is becoming more conscious of the areas that need to be changed. I think, if nothing else, people are looking at it hard and they're doing things to cut their expenses. That's got to be good in the long run.

On a national basis, California, the Northwest and the Northeast are definitely the trend setters. While most of the nation has been waiting to see what Clinton's going to do, these areas started to act in anticipation of what's going to happen, regardless of whether it's right or wrong. From what I've witnessed, the rest of the country is not participating in this managed-care trend. They're going to have a rude awakening because they haven't pared down enough. The medical industry in some areas is relatively healthy from a cost overrun standpoint. But some parts of the country—it's incredible, just incredible. In my travels from headquarters it just amazes me what I see. They're like ostriches in the sand.

C an we take care of all the people that are going to come into the system? I think the system can handle a lot more than it does. I don't know if we've got the correct systems in place to do it. Maybe it isn't the emergency room that's needed, it might be the nurse practitioner. It's a redistribution of resources. With that in mind we can increase quality and decrease costs.

O ur country has been based on a capitalistic, free market model that has worked very well for quite some time. I think we would all agree that what has happened in the socialist, communist countries in the last ten years shows the superiority that is inherent in a free market system where the individual is rewarded commensurate with his effort. As soon as you take that away, you develop a system where mediocrity is the rule. I'm afraid the road we're heading down in health care is a road to mediocrity.

I see nothing positive coming of government stepping in to solve our health-care problems. I see it as entirely negative. The government has already proved that they're incompetent at administrating virtually everything, especially health care. The Veterans Administration system is probably the best example. They've been running entire hospitals, entire purchasing departments for many, many years. The quality of service is low. The consumer who uses their service is dissatisfied with it. Ask anyone who's required to go to the VA hospital for treatment. If they had the choice between going there and going to another hospital, which would they choose? I bet in nearly every case, they would choose not to go to the VA. That should say it all.

You know we do draw a lot of foreign people who have money who want to come here because we have a good health-care system. We draw a lot of Canadians. Totally revamping the system when it's only a little bit broken doesn't make any sense to me, but that's what the current administration wants to do.

Access to health care? We all have access to health care. Maybe not our ideal vision of what we want, but we already all have access. If you're really sick, all you have to do is show up at a hospital. Any hospital you want. You can't be refused treatment. It's against the law. You may get transferred to the county hospital, but you'll still be treated. They may put you on a cash payment plan, but you won't be thrown out the door to die in the gutter if you don't have the right card in your wallet. I really don't understand why they keep promoting this idea that there's this huge sector of our population that has absolutely no health care available to them. It's bullshit. True, certain areas like preventive care may be limited or nonexistent, but if you or I had a heart attack this minute, if the paramedics could get here in time, we would be treated regardless of whether we had insurance or not.

I think one of the greatest influences on the final outcome of health-care reform lies with the news media. Although they claim to be objective and only reporting the facts, they don't always get the facts right. And they also look for the most sensational aspect of whatever they're reporting on. I think the Clintons know this and have played it quite well to their advantage.

I really think the American people are getting a distorted view of the health-care industry because the press put so much emphasis on public opinion polls. This in turn influences our politicians who are looking to get the vote in the next election. And suddenly, we're driven by the opinion of the general public, a group that really doesn't have the faintest idea about how the health-care industry really works. They're just reacting to what they read and hear and see in the media. So it all gets back to the news media.

M edia and advertising. Two things that distort the truth. For instance, we always hear the study that comes out that is the most inflammatory. We never hear the fact that it was a poorly designed study, it was rejected by another study that followed it up. We don't hear that as a nation. The media keep coming out with these little blurbs, and the nation has gotten confused. You tell a patient something and they say, "But I just read. . . ." The media and advertising confuse them, and so sometimes people just throw up their hands and say, "Oh, well."

One of the best ways to improve our health care is to ignore the media and advertising.

T hey should get rid of a system like Medicaid that allows emergency room treatment for anything and everything. Where, if a patient came into our ER with a nonthreatening problem, we could refer them to a clinic next door. They would probably cut their costs billions of dollars in our state alone even if they just had Medicaid clinics open.

W ill it be that you and I will have this mediocre system to deal with, but the president and the people in government will have special treatment? If you look at the track record of other countries, I wouldn't be surprised.

I think reform is going to be healthy from what I hear so far. Anytime you can get to a point where you're providing a service to everybody and it's on a cost effective continuum, sounds wonderful to me. I don't worry as so many of my colleagues do about it because I'm not in an area where I can make a lot of money.

T here's a certain amount of entrepreneurship that's necessary in health care or it will stagnate. You can regulate them. You can control their profits. But they need a certain amount of incentive capital to make it worth their while. Unless we want medicine to stagnate as it has in Europe and Canada.

People think medicine is great in Europe and Canada because they don't have to pay for anything. It's not. You have to wait seven months to have a cataract operation in Canada. You could be blind by that time and then it won't do any good. But they don't care because that's the type of system that was created.

You talk to ten different people, they give you ten different answers right now. The consensus is that there's no way to tell, because what the president wants has still got to pass through Congress, and they'll have massaged that thing in such a fashion that it will probably be quite different by the time it passes. The lobbyists haven't had their shot at it yet, either. There's no way to tell what it's going to end up like.

It will be interesting. The problem is, no one knows the rules and until you know what the rules are, you can't figure out where you're going to land—on your feet or on your head. No one will know until it's done. Once the rules are known, there's always ways around them, there's always gaps to find and everybody will fit in and settle into it.

I'm not real optimistic about health-care reform. Having a private office, I'm not sure how it's going to affect me. Plus, being a small business, I'm not sure what the tax situation is going to be. I'm afraid that small businesses like mine are going to carry the brunt of funding the insurance. We can't afford that. I'm barely paying my payroll taxes on time.

I'm not sure if we're all going to be drawn into a large HMO kind of clinic. I'm not sure how the gatekeeper system is going to work for private practices. I just have a lot of questions and I haven't seen any answers really.

If the politicians want to legislate reform, fine, then let's do it and get it done and get on with our lives.

I n my business, most physicians are afraid of managed care because they don't know what the impact is going to be. They're
sitting back, not buying, not hiring. They're just hanging around
just to see what the impact is going to be. So the guy who last year
told me that this year he was going to spend $60,000 for a ma-
chine, isn't buying this year either. He's still waiting to see what's
going to happen.

T he health reform package will probably go the route of all
tax reform. When it's finally signed, sealed and delivered, it
won't be much different than it is now.

B ecause the solution to our problems in health care disem-
powers both politicians and insurance companies, it will
never happen. That's the sad reality of what we're faced with.
The politicians who thrive on power are not going to give it up,
and the insurance companies with $2 trillion worth of assets
aren't about to give it up either.

I looked Clinton's plan over, and I think it does have some good
points, but I am leery of government in any way, shape or form
taking control of anything. And if you don't think they're going
to take control because they say they're not going to, don't believe
it. In 1933 or whenever Social Security was first started, Roosevelt
promised the American people if they would support his social
security program the most they would ever pay—ever—is one half
of one percent. We know where that promise went—up over fifteen percent.

In the mid-sixties when LBJ and his Great Society was going
to wipe out poverty, you know how well that went. When they
started the Medicare program, he projected that the most it would
cost by 1990 was maybe $6 billion or $7 billion. He was off by a
factor of ten. Whenever you have the government going to solve
a problem, they invariably make it worse. I'm afraid what we have
here is that kind of scenario.

I know the concept of national health care, to make health care available to everyone, but I think that health care is going to be limited. Not all services will be available to everyone. At what point do you say no? That's going to raise a lot of issues for patients and families. Why is one entitled when the other isn't?

You have to be very careful as to what age you start rationing care. I do think we have to educate the populace that if you have had a cardiac arrest and are eighty-five years old, it's pointless to try to save you. What would your life be like? You're not going to be twenty years old again. You may live another year or so but it's going to be a miserable existence. When it's time to go, we should be allowed to go. This is one of those real touchy issues. At what age then do you start cutting people off?

Reform begins with educating the public as to how to take care of themselves. To educate the public in terms of what's available in their community and how to utilize it. Then, teaching them how to communicate their wishes and know that they have rights, and they have rights to express those wishes to their physician, their hospital, whoever they interface with.

Educating the public, too, in terms of when enough is enough. For instance, do we use our health-care dollars, sometimes hundreds of thousands of dollars, to maintain someone who has no quality of life on a machine and will never have any more than that? Do we take those dollars away from someone who has a chance for recovery? I understand that these are very difficult questions. Some people say, "I want everything done, no matter what my quality of life is." But as taxpayers, paying those dollars out to someone who's eighty-five or ninety years old who is on a ventilator and in a coma or a vegetative state and will never walk out of the hospital, does that patient or family have the right to demand that our health-care dollars be spent on that person?

I'd say, looking at an average of a hundred patients, maybe ten percent exhaust the dollars from that ninety percent. If you have a limited amount of dollars spent on health care, and eighty-five percent of those dollars is going toward that ten percent, it exhausts what's available to the rest of the ninety percent. That's what's happened to our health care, so much of the dollar amount has been exhausted on the concept of futile care. This is raising lots of issues of looking at quality of life, effective medicine, medicine that becomes futile, and being comfortable with stopping futile treatment.

O ur company gives great service and accurate results. Say that I charge fifty bucks [to the doctor] and the doctor then charges $300 to $400. He orders the test and signs his name to the report and takes the responsibility if there's a problem. How much is that worth? Three hundred and fifty dollars? Who determines what's fair? Some government agency? I don't like that. If they dictate what the doctor can charge, it won't be long before they do the same to me. I'm in business to make a profit, and I don't want some bureaucrat deciding how much I deserve to make on my work.

T here are new EKG machines that are computerized and perform interpretive functions. Until recently, reimbursement for an EKG was broken down into a technical component and an interpretation fee. If the hospital does the EKG with their equipment and their staff, they get twenty bucks or so. That's the technical component. The doctor who then reads the test could also charge for his part and receive the interpretation fee.

Well, a bunch of politicians were given the statistics and they said, "Look at how much money these doctors are making off interpreting EKGs. Tell you what, now that some computerized EKG machines have the capacity to interpret the test, the doctor doesn't even have to read it anymore. Why should he get reimbursed for interpretation?" So what do they do? They decided not to give doctors reimbursement rates for reading EKGs anymore.

This shows again how stupid politicians are. Computers are great tools for all of us to use, but they're not the final answer to everything. Computers still can be fooled. You can't always get a technically good EKG. If you've got a little old patient lying in bed shaking from fear or medication or whatever, or if you have an obese patient, most of the time you're not going to get a test that a computer can interpret correctly. You still need a doctor to verify the accuracy of the computer's interpretation.

But the government can't understand that because they're not in the field performing the tests. They just look at the dollar bottom line and make decisions. In doing so, they took the whole EKG business and put it in the toilet for the last two years, and I think have markedly decreased the quality of care as well.

I understand that reimbursement for interpretations is coming back next year, because they've realized they've made a mistake—another good example of how inept bureaucrats and politicians are in making health-care decisions.

I don't believe the components of Clinton's plan need to be a push toward socialized medicine, but when you have the health-care alliances, which are going to be huge—bigger than any other segment of government because of the number of dollars that go through those things—that will create a huge bureaucracy. And in quite rapid fashion, I think we would be into a socialized system.

I don't think the Clinton reform plan would last long. Because of the cost problems, it would rapidly move into a Canadian style, single-payer system. The government would be the payer, and that would be it. You would negotiate only with the government. I think that kills a lot of the good that's in our system now of opportunity to experiment and test and develop things more efficiently and effectively.

Let's build the system. Let's get the counterproductive laws out of the way and provide a mechanism so that we can provide care more effectively. Give patients an incentive to buy the most efficient type of health care instead of the luxury of the fee-for-service. First-dollar coverage is a travesty, it's a real noose around our necks. We don't need that kind of coverage, it's buying the wrong kind of health care.

M y primary area of activity, both statewide and nationally, has been in working on public policy issues and strategies for health care in the future.

I don't think "crisis" is the right word to describe where we're at in health care today. If it is the right word, then we've always been in a crisis. I see health care as having been for a good many years in a state of evolution, and I think it will continue. If the Clinton reform package does happen to get passed, which I don't think will happen, that will only be another step in this continuing evolution of change.

At the moment, we are evolving into a process whereby the providers of health care will be better aligned with the same in-centives to provide care efficiently—that's what will happen under a capitation payment. They're going to be paid for taking care of umpteen number of patients, and whether the patient costs more or less, that's the money they get. That helps on the efficiency side.

Capitation has been taking place long before Clinton ever came up with the proposal, and will whether any of his proposals are introduced or not.

T aking the country as a whole, the general public definitely does not have realistic expectations of what our health-care system can and should provide for them. They say, "yes we need health-care reform," because they've read that some people, thir-ty-seven million perhaps, don't have health care. It's not them, it's not us, but they've read about it and seen all these scenes of people who don't get proper care, and said, "That's terrible."

But the general public is not ready for the fact that in order to take care of that group, this main group has to give up something, and in fact has to give up a lot. It will cost them more. Their access to care will be curtailed.

T he federal government is the problem in health care. There's mismanagement, way too much paperwork, way too much waste, the service cost is too high. For example, we have three outpatient areas that do mammography. Medicare pays us—very little money—for screening mammograms, but they also want us to go through this long audit trail. We had five people spend an entire week scrambling around, answering questions and filling out forms. But if you don't do it, they won't pay. By law we have to do it.

The College of Radiology has one set of requirements, the state has another set of requirements, and Medicare has a different set, so if you satisfy one, you may not satisfy another. But if you don't satisfy everybody, you won't get paid. It's a matter of economics. It just gets worse every year; and it changes every year.

What do we need to do to reform health care? Boy, I guess if I had the answer to that I'd be sitting in the White House. I think universal health care for everybody is a real good idea. I don't think anybody knows exactly how to do it because it's so large.

I want to know, how's it going to be paid for? If it goes to national health care and everybody's going to be covered, how are they going to do it? Somebody's going to have to pay. I know I've heard that we're going to pay for it by the savings we'll realize when government steps in and forces things to run more efficiently. To me, that's a conflict of terms. Have you ever heard of one government program that is known to run efficiently? Have you ever heard of one instance where the government stepped in and made things run smoother? Hasn't bureaucracy become synonymous with inefficiency?

That leaves one other solution: raise taxes.

If everybody starts putting money in a pool for insurance, from the outset you're going to have billions of dollars in the hands of somebody. Who's going to control it? The same people who put this country $3 trillion in debt? We've got the government wanting to come in and control costs, to determine the bottom line. Looking at their track record, it's not too hard to predict the outcome of that.

I don't think we need to have "shopping center" medicine. We don't need a CAT scanner on every corner. But I do think that as long as we've got this technology and ability, people should have access to it.

Since we got started in our business back in 1978, we've had a medical plan that is as good as or better than any other on the market. I want my people to have better care and it's hard core business sense, because I'm much more competitive as far as keeping my employees with that kind of a plan. It works both ways. I get repaid for it. I'm afraid that Clinton is going to change that, I'm afraid that it's going to diminish the quality of insurance I have for myself and my employees.

I was working in the hospital when Medicare came into effect. I see the same thing happening with Hillary's health-care reform bill.

Before Medicare started, I was working in the radiology department of a major hospital, we used to go into shock when we would have to do exams on anybody over fifty years old. We just didn't see a lot of old people. And the day Medicare went into effect, it was like somebody opened up the floodgates from all the retirement communities in the area. We suddenly had people in their eighties and nineties coming in because, basically, it was free. They would say, "Yeah, I haven't had a checkup in forty years. I think I'll just have it all done now." The doctors were delighted to write the orders for all the money they'd be making.

There's always some way to get around anything.

The first step in meaningful reform would be to wring the waste out of the existing system.

The current American health-care system is sick, but it is not terminally ill. The political concern is with costs, not quality.

Granted, a large segment of our population is uninsured and that is a social disgrace, but that deficiency can be corrected without destroying the best medical care the world has ever known.

National health-care reform is a product of two fundamental problems with the current medical delivery system and insurance industry. One, the seemingly uncontrollable rising health-care costs. And two, the alleged lack of health insurance for a significant number of Americans. I don't think anyone will argue the validity of the first. The second, however, doesn't appear as certain. Has anyone heard exactly how they arrived at that huge number? Who are they counting as uninsured?

There's intense interest in solving America's health-care crisis, but it extends far beyond the moral dilemma that our current system excludes 37 million people. The reform that envisions universal access to health services will create a system that will prevent universal use of the system. Yes, you could have theoretical access to medical care, but the bureaucracy would limit your using the available medical services.

There's a group of people in this Catch-22 that don't have health insurance. They're in a job that doesn't offer medical benefits. They're part-time and work thirty hours a week and make seven bucks an hour. They can't turn around and pay $400 or $500 a month for medical insurance, and they make too much to be on welfare. Those are the people that don't have medical care and that are just cash every time they walk in. They're the ones I'm worried about.

The basis of the Clinton plan is universal coverage, paid largely by employers, and delivered through a system of budgeted managed competition. This approach falls somewhere between a regulated, socialized, single-payer approach, and free-enterprise, free-market competition. Managed care has been wrongly identified with free-market views. The truth is that managed care with its global budgets involves plenty of regulation. When nations throughout the world are abandoning maximum government central planning, why are we taking up a philosophy that has failed for others?

The irony of the reform package is that it appears to be anti-insurance industry, but it isn't. If implemented, the insurance companies through their HMOs will have your money anyway, and your health will not be the prime objective.

Fortunately, the Clinton health-care plan will never be implemented. Somewhere between sixty and seventy Democrat members of the House of Representatives are firmly committed to the single-payer, Canadian, system. They represent congressional districts where the majority of voters expect that kind of health-care delivery system. Those advocates for the Canadian system would jeopardize their chances for re-election if they voted for the Clinton plan. So the president must negotiate with the Republicans. With national elections in 1994, does anyone believe for one moment that the political opposition is going to help the president? There might be a bipartisan attempt to develop universal access to the health-care delivery system, but it will take many, many years.

There is no cure for health care in the Clinton plan. It's a shell game. Managed competition in health care is going to cost everybody dearly. The Clinton administration wants to turn over fourteen percent of the GNP to something called managed competition in the hope that the marketplace will become a vehicle for social policy. There is a great irony in all of this. For years the Republicans have talked of free market economics, now it is the New Democrats who are attempting to institutionalize it. The United States now spends much more on health: $2,500 annually for every American, against Canada's $1,800 and the United Kingdom's $1,000. Since all Western countries are affected by the same types and rates of illnesses, it is generally thought that the basic problem is the very private insurance system that President Clinton would preserve by giving it a monopoly.

T he HMO system will be a bare bones policy of benefits. The Clinton plan takes money from the Medicaid program with an overhead of three percent and will shift it to the private insurance system which currently has an overhead of thirteen percent. The rationale of the plan is to squeeze the savings out of the providers, not out of patients. The problem is that providers are a more powerful group than the patients.

M anaged care will change the insurance industry by putting it in the hands of a few large companies which have already invested heavily in HMOs. If the Clinton plan is enacted, a few insurance companies will own and control the system. Then the call for the breakup of the monopoly will be the political-social issue of national politics.

I have an insurance plan that covers me and my family—there's five of us. I'm forty-five years old, my wife turns forty next month. This insurance plan costs us $178 per month. Very reasonable. I have a $2,000 deductible. I have to pay the first $2,000 out of my pocket—doctor's visits, prescriptions, dentist appointments, and so forth. This way I shop around for quality and price. If the doctor is too high, I'll make a few phone calls. If the prescription is too high, I'll make a few phone calls. I will find the place that provides me with the quality of service that I expect, and I'll pay a reasonable price for it.

If something tragic happens, like I develop bone cancer, I know that I'm going to get the proper tests to see what's wrong. I have to pay my initial $2,000, and then I have to pay twenty percent of the next $5,000, which is another $1,000. So if I'm in the hospital ringing up a $300,000 bill, I pay $3,000. For $178 a month.

What we have to get the people in this country used to is once again paying for their own health care. Everyone in the country could have the best health care that they want at a reasonable price, if you get the insurance company the hell out of the way. If you get them back into providing insurance and not dictating the health-care marketplace, you'll stop the price fixing that they're imposing on all of us, you'll stop the red tape that they're tying us up with, you'll stop the market collusion and the market allocation practices they're engaged in, you'll stcp the coercion of the patient to trade at providers of the insurance company's choice, not the patient's choice.

So the true solution is this. Number one. You keep the politicians the hell away from health care. Health care is much too serious an issue to get the politicians involved in. Keep them away. Let them foul up the post office or whatever, but not health care. Number two, you get the insurance companies the hell out of managing health care and you let the patients choose.

That will work. It has all the basics in it. It has the patient making the choice, the marketplace fixing the prices and level of service, and everyone is protected against catastrophic loss. What more could you want?

T he continuing rise in health-care expenditures contributes to America's weakening international competitive position. Nearly half of real per capita income gains over the past decade has been spent on satisfying the nation's insatiable health-care appetite. As a result, it's been diverting monies from other critical needs such as education, crime prevention, housing, transportation, industrial revival and research.

In two years, health-care costs will reach nearly $1 trillion, representing sixteen percent of the entire US economy. By the year 2000, in six years, without intervention, health-care costs are estimated to rise to about twenty percent of the economy. Without cost containment and cost reduction, the health-care delivery system will diminish the financial and human resource investment opportunities of our nation. If a cure is not found now, the United States will become a second-rate economic power. The health, welfare and financial well-being of our nation hangs in the balance. The future of our country's ten million employers, 600,000 physicians, 6,000 hospitals, three million other health-care professionals and every single American and their offspring for generations to come is in jeopardy.

14

PATIENTS' RIGHTS—AND RESPONSIBILITIES

The absolute bottom line in health care, both in terms of costs and quality of life always was, and always will be, the patient.

The health-care professionals we spoke with are committed to providing the highest quality care possible, but many also voiced a strong desire to see patients assume an equal share of responsibility for their own health. Health care, they told us, is more than surgery, drug therapy, hospitalization or office visits—it is lifestyle. First and foremost, health care is taught and practiced in the home. We can thoroughly understand the frustration of the health-care professional when a patient comes to them and says, "I've made a mess of my body. You do something about it for me. I don't have the time, or the desire, to take care of it myself."

What we want people to do is to not use the system to an excess. That's why the old-fashioned major deductibles make sense. If I have to spend the first $1,000 of my own money, with that $1,000 that I take out of my pocket, I'm going to spend that as intelligently as I can because that's my money. Then, after it gets to a thousand dollars I'll say, "Well that's the insurance company's money." Then I'll be frivolous with it.

If you have first-dollar coverage, where the insurance company is going to pay for the very first dollar you spend on health care, you're going to buy a lot more health care than if it was coming out of your own pocket.

What people don't realize is, it is coming out of your own pocket—you're paying it in a monthly premium. The delusion is that your employer is paying that. No, no. You are paying it. You would have gotten more money in your paycheck if your employer wasn't paying that insurance premium for you.

Yet, the idea that you're getting a free lunch because somebody else is paying for it is pervasive now. Most people think that health care will be free. It is not and never will be. One way or another, you will be paying for it. If the government takes it over, it will not be free. You're going to pay for it in taxes or whatever system they come up with, and it will still be very expensive.

If something is free, it's always overutilized. The smartest guy in the world is the guy who's spending his own money. The whole health-care system will run better if we can get that idea across to the consumer. You, the consumer, are the best one to decide how your dollar gets spent. Because whether you know it or not, it's your dollar.

According to public opinion polls, a majority of Americans are satisfied with their current coverage, but fear losing their jobs and thus their health coverage. People want all of the health care that's available and are demanding impossible assurances that coverage and benefits will not be reduced, that there will be coverage for everyone, free choice of services and little or no cost increase to pay for it. With that kind of thinking, it won't be long before we start suing the government every time we get sick. And winning!

Most people that I deal with realize that if you're going to get quality health care, you're going to have to pay for it. It's like anything else in life. You get what you pay for. If you expect somebody to give you something for free, you're going to get exactly what you paid for.

T he education program is impossible. You cannot educate 200 million people that it's their dollar. Somehow, they will still think it's somebody else's dollar being spent. It's going to be some rich person who's paying some exorbitant amount of tax who's going to take care of me. Or it's going to be a middle class worker because I'm retired now so I don't have any income, so I don't pay any income taxes and it's free. No. One way or another, it has to get paid for. You can't just print up more doctors. You can't pass a law and suddenly create more health care. The pie's only so big, and if you get twice the utilization, all the pieces of pie are half as big. Rationed health care is going to happen.

N ot only do people think they have a right to health care, but if there is anything out there, if there is any kind of a device, if there is any kind of a procedure, if there is any form of intervention that might just give them a marginal improvement in their quality of life or expectation of life, then they think they're entitled to that. That's the definition of health care. We can't afford that definition.

In the Clinton plan—if we go through with it—the economic pieces are in place to start ratcheting down the amount of money that's available. What's not clearly in place is how you change the expectations of people.

If you were a restaurant owner and ten years ago you decided to make your restaurant a smoke-free restaurant, everybody would have said, "You're crazy. You'll go out of business." Today, if you look what's happened over the last ten years or so through this gradual process of education, that pattern is now socially acceptable. There are still some die-hard smokers who don't like it, but they recognize that they are outside the mainstream of society today, whereas ten or fifteen years ago, when the percentage of people who smoked was higher, they felt they had the right to smoke whenever and wherever they pleased. So we have definitely changed society's expectations of a certain set of actions. We need to do exactly the same thing with regard to health care.

T here's a certain segment that insists health care is a right and somebody, somewhere should give it to them. Those people have no concept of what a right actually is, and they have no idea of who this somebody is that's going to provide it for them. If you're going to get something for nothing, that you're not paying for, well someone else is.

A right is something such as the right to free speech. You can say what you want, and it doesn't make me pay you any money or provide you with a service or provide you with a product. Once you demand something like health care as a right, now you're saying that I owe you something. I, the health-care provider, because I'm a health-care provider, I am now obligated to give you something for which I'm not going to be compensated. That used to be called thievery.

How can an individual cut down his or her cost of health care? What it really gets down to are the basics. Number one, attention to not only good health but sensible lifestyle practices. Getting into the habit of using seat belts. Getting into the habit of good diet. Getting into the habit of good exercise and keeping yourself reasonably fit. Not smoking, avoiding alcohol or other things that are bad for you.

Your mental view of this is key. I'm fascinated with the studies done on holistic medicine and mental forms of healing, which is not to say physical conditions are nonexistent, but there's lots of interesting research that shows that a positive mental attitude can really improve the healing process. We do a lot of things to ourselves because we are mad at ourselves or our self-image is poor.

The other thing that we can do is educate ourselves on how to recognize real conditions from minor conditions. There are a number of books out that in addition to talking about good nutrition and all, it basically gives sort of a home primer on first aid and recognizing the conditions that are self-limiting, recognizing what conditions are such that you ought to seek professional care, and what are fairly routine and don't really require that level of intervention. All of those forms of education are critical.

And, of course, bringing your children up in that same way. Raising your children in an environment that tries to get away from this sense of entitlement, makes them feel that they are responsible for their own actions.

One of the large public utility companies in our area, for example, a few years ago introduced four lifestyle questions in the annual open enrollment in its health-care plan. These had to do with not smoking, low alcohol usage, normal weight, blood pressure. If you could answer yes to those four questions, they would give a small reduction in the premium that you paid in your health insurance. It was not an actuarial equivalent premium, but they were trying to start creating this image which said, what we as an employer are paying for the health care of our employees is less for those people that are healthier. You the employee needs to recognize that and we'll share a little bit of that with you. Your costs should be less as well.

M y grandmother died of leukemia because they overradiated her after a mastectomy in a small town in southern Minnesota. Do you think my parents would sue the hospital? No, that hospital was the lifeblood of that community. They were proud of it, they wouldn't do it. Today, litigation is as much a part of our health-care system as doctors and nurses.

It's because our expectations have gotten so great. I suppose it started with President Johnson's idea of the Great Society and all these wonderful things that we're supposed to get. And the next thing you know, you had carpeting down the halls in the hospital, and you had to expect that a nurse would answer your bell within a few minutes. The attitude was more of a "take care of me." We suddenly had elderly coming into the hospital when their family got tired of taking care of them. We'd take care of them for a week or two and then they'd go home. That was sort of the way things became. We started to overuse everything. We overused it to the max because it was paid for.

I remember when my kids were little. We lived in Colorado, and the local Blue Cross recognized that wellness care would eventually pay off, so there was first-dollar coverage for everything. Of course within a couple of years they had to stop it. They couldn't afford the cost. It encouraged people, but without the education or the sense of responsibility.

P revention is an area that is not well understood. Families and individuals often don't know what prevention is. They see prevention as an immunization and that's it. They don't see life-style changes and how necessary that is and what that means. Somehow, just as when you're driving and you get a ticket and there's a way that you can get that remedied by going to driving classes, there ought to be a requirement that the individual go to class and show evidence that they're trying to make some change, if they are to continue to get health-care delivery.

There's got to be some hard decisions made like that, and I think those lie primarily in changing health-care behavior, in prevention. That's where the greatest emphasis goes.

I owned a diagnostic service that was a testing facility. Testing, in and of itself, is good. If the American people had the opportunity to have more tests done on themselves at a price that was more reasonable, I don't see a problem with that. The problem is we can't afford it as a nation. Not everyone can have every test they desire and claim it's their right.

J ust because a patient wants something, that doesn't mean they're necessarily going to get it. It's becoming our job to help people to understand the allocation of resources and the inevitable fact that we're moving in that direction. The medical society in general has to begin to accept limiting those resources as well. We can't do everything for everybody. It's very frustrating, because if that was your son or your daughter or your mother or your father, you would want everything done if it might be beneficial. But that may not necessarily be the case anymore.

T here's no question that all of us want the best technology to be used that will help people to get well, but on the other hand, one of the great problems in health care today is that nobody wants to bite the bullet and say, "I really don't think this procedure is necessary for the patient. It's very necessary for my research. It's very necessary for the hospital's revenue or even my own personal income, but it's not for the patient." The families themselves don't want to take the responsibility of saying, "Would you please stop now? This person is eighty or ninety years old, and I do not want their life extended."

You don't see the caretakers wanting to make decisions either. They often will say, "Well, you do what is right. You tell me what should be done." I think frankly that we as health professionals need to address these families in a meaningful way and say, "As far as I am concerned, for the patient's good, this is what I think would be best." It's very difficult to get nurses, families, or doctors to come to grips with it, and I see more of a tendency today for the physicians and nurses and the whole group, wanting to put that decision on the family.

At the time of impending death, that's not the time to make the patient or the family have to come up with a decision. They need to give some preliminary directives, that's important. But they need to do that in a time of wellness. Then that needs to be supported and guided through by the medical team.

A Durable Power of Attorney, or a Living Will, is essential. It should be dealt with early in life, and should not wait until the person is in their senior years. It needs to be reviewed at different stages through life. An eighteen year old is not too young at all to think, "How do I wish to die?" I don't want to die now, but if some major episode happened to me and my life was at stake, these are the decisions that I would like to be able to have a part of, and this is how I would like to decide." That component then needs to be reviewed every few years until that person is no longer able to review it.

We're looking at various policies in terms of patient care, and not specific issues, but in terms of things like Durable Power of Attorney for health care. Part of our role has been to help implement and develop an education program. I believe it was 1976 when our state introduced the Natural Death Act. Eventually it evolved into the Patient Self-Determination Act, which allows a patient to complete, when they are alert, awake and oriented, a Durable Power of Attorney for health care. It's a form which if a patient were to become incapacitated or unable to make their own decisions, it allows them to appoint someone to make those decisions for them. It allows them to express their wishes as to what they would want done, whether it would be to terminate life support, whether it would be to provide all the possible care available to them, whether they would want organ donation or no organ donation, or anything specifically related to their health care in general.

This is something that is good indefinitely unless you add an expiration date to it. It's something that doesn't necessarily have to be notarized. It can be. If it's not notarized, it has to be signed by two people who know that you're doing this without being under duress, and that the two people who witness it cannot be one of your appointed agents and cannot be named in your will or have any benefit to gain from you.

It's something that we're stressing more and more. I know recently Bill and Hillary filled one out. Sometimes they're called Living Wills. In our state we refer to them as Durable Power of Attorney for Health Care. We encourage a patient to fill one out now while they're well and able, then give a copy to their physician. If they have to go to the hospital, the hospital should have a copy. And give one to their agent, whether it be a son or daughter, sister or brother, parent, a friend—it can be anybody. And finally, carry a copy in your wallet, to show that you have one.

I'm a young person and I've completed a Durable Power of Attorney for health care. I could be hit by a car tomorrow and I've now communicated my wishes. We're encouraging not only the elderly but the young. You have to be eighteen and over to complete one. And if at anytime you choose to disregard what you've done, all you have to do is rip it up or fill out a new one, and the new one takes the place.

W e all want the best. We all want the Cadillac. But is the Cadillac necessary to get us to the store? It could be a VW or lesser. An old, old, old VW would be adequate. I am very much opposed to the government paying for the Cadillac system.

I do believe that health is a right. I believe that the vast majority of us are willing to pay for the bare essentials for life and health support, including emergency pickup of individuals who are in accidents, et cetera. That would include a certain level of preventive services. It would include basic health care. Then the question is, what is basic? But it would not include the broad technological advances that we now have that are extremely costly.

Quite frankly, in all the health-care packages that I've seen, I would tend to lean more toward the Oregonian method. Like, how much money can we spend? How much money do we have? And then buy the best that we possibly can. But don't say, "Let's all aim at getting new Cadillacs for all of our children." That's really ridiculous.

At the same time we need to have a collective look, administratively, in health care, at how much is needed for research; how much is needed for general health care; how much money then can we provide? Help citizens know that it's going to cost dearly, but this is what we're going to pay for. We're going to pay for a level of prevention. We'll pay for the first episodes of whatever, but that's all we're going to pay for. You're going to have to help us make some of the hard decisions. If there is no more government money to pay for your second bypass, or pay for a bypass after a certain age.

It's a very difficult thing for a hospital or an insurance company to say to you, "We're not going to pay for your father's heart surgery because he's seventy-two years old. He's got a bad heart history. His chances of survival are only ten or twenty percent. We would expend a hundred thousand dollars in resources. That's a hundred thousand dollars of resources that we could use to take care of the prenatal care of five hundred women, or the basic nutritional needs of some other large number of people." But ultimately we're going to come down to that.

People have a very hard time dealing with that. They say,

"How can you put dollar value on human life? He's entitled to that. I'm entitled to that." And yet, if you didn't have insurance, and you had to sell everything you had to do that, there are some people who would just make that knee-jerk reaction, that emotional response and say, "Yes. I'll do it." I suspect that with a little bit of education, if you could bring people around to saying, "Is this expenditure of resources worth the outcome?" you would begin to change some of that thought process. I think it has to change.

We had a case where a patient was very sick and had several surgeries that proved to be ineffective. The family continued to want everything done. He ended up developing a significant infection, was on a ventilator, was unresponsive, and ended up having all kinds of horrible things oozing from his body. His family continued to want everything done. The doctors were uncomfortable. He was just riddled with infection. His family still wanted everything done.

The man went into cardiac arrest and they had to pump on his chest. It was just so traumatic for the nurses because he had absolutely no dignity, no quality, and was really being brutalized. And the family still wanted everything done. After about ten weeks of this, he finally passed on. I feel that the patient went through some real agony and some real injustice at the family's not wanting to let go. This patient was clearly suffering. It was real difficult for all of us because we wanted to let this man have some dignity and some grace, and we couldn't.

I am a good example. I'm a nurse and also have gone through the system myself. I was born with an aortic valvular problem. I had an aortic valve replacement to the tune of about $70,000 for that package about six years ago. My insurance paid the big bulk of that. My question then, ethically, is, should every person in society be ready to pay for a $70,000 cardiac procedure? It extends life. Life is good. I hope that I've contributed a lot and have a lot to go. I think I would say, well the first time, prior to sixty, maybe yes. But I would definitely say, absolutely not the second time. I know many individuals who have gone in to have a second runaround with another valve. Somewhere a line has to be drawn.

Now if I personally choose to have a second valve, then that's my choice, but I've got to help raise the money then. I've got to raise it through my whole united family and come to grips with the fact that there isn't any more money. Frankly, I don't think that would be too hard for me to say, "No, this is not economically sound. It isn't smart at all." Yet, I know many, many, many individuals who have gotten second, third, fourth bypasses. At tremendous costs. And I know many that were at the end of life anyway, and have not had a bettered life after those bypasses. To me, that is uncalled for.

I would say that in the majority of cases we spend our dollars on the other end of the spectrum, where we could probably do much better service if we started earlier. Quality of care should include what you prevent as well as how you treat it once it's happened.

The Clinton speech that kicked off his health-care reform package, it was like "fairy tale city," him saying it's not going to cost us that much more. The cost of all of this is going to be tremendous because you're going to have people accessing the medical system that have never accessed it before. It's a shame that they haven't been able to, but now when they're able to, they will.

So now you're going to hear everyone saying, "It's my right to have this and that." And they're going to want the best that the system has to offer. That's not unreasonable. But if we have all the more people demanding the best service, the system won't be able to provide that. The quality will drop for all. I mean, we're stretched as it is here at this hospital. It's like blowing more people into this balloon called health care. It's already stretched taut. I'm afraid that forcing more into it will cause it to pop, and it's going to explode with a bang.

We need a financial incentive for people to take responsibility for their own health care. There has not been a financial incentive for—I'm going to call them "the poor" but I would say up into the middle class. The people who are on Medicaid are individuals who are in our welfare systems. Those individuals have come to the place where they are dependent upon the system, and they are expecting the system to fix everything. They really couldn't care less about caring for themselves. Somebody has to nurture their own abilities to care and show them the reason why it is better to care for themselves. Somehow, we've got to help get that point across more.

At this point, they see other role models—their parents who have treated them like that, where if they had the sniffles their parents went and told some doctor at an emergency room, "I think my child is getting pneumonia." Make the issue big and it will be cared for; otherwise, it won't be. They're willing to go through the waiting for that, even though they complain about it. That's what they've been raised to do.

If a patient walks into an emergency room with an HMO insurance, and it's for something stupid, his insurance provider is going to deny treatment. Medicaid patients are never denied treatment at all. I had a woman come in with a bruise on a finger. You're talking a $200 charge to be told she had a bruised finger.

Simple colds. We are constantly seeing them. You have the parents saying, "Jaime, here, has a runny nose. I'm going to take him to the emergency room. And, well, these two are kind of sniffling a little so I better take them too." We call it the family plan. The whole family will be seen. All five people will come in. You're talking at least $100 emergency room visit charge and $100 doctor charge per individual. So this family walks in, and an hour later Medicaid owes the hospital $1,000 for one child with a cold.

Here our state is already in a terrible financial crisis, and we have Medicaid people just walking into an emergency room saying, "I've had a side ache for a month." We ask, "You didn't think to go to your doctor?" And they say, "I don't have a doctor."

Fifty percent of those who come to the emergency room, don't have doctors, regular physicians, so they bop into the hospital emergency room every single time they want treatment.

A child will come in with a runny nose and a sore throat, and the mom will be expecting an antibiotic. They don't know that most clear runny noses are viral infections and antibiotics won't help. Sure, sometimes antibiotics can be used if this is a chronic kid who's liable to get something else from it, but the antibiotics are to given to prevent something else from developing, not to cure the runny nose. But these moms come in already knowing what they want.

Parents need education in what is what. Our viruses and bacteria are changing all the time too. A raw throat could be bacterial where an antibiotic wouldn't help, but we'll treat it anyway, because if you don't, this mom is going to be back a day later because that sore throat hasn't gone away. You're going to possibly give that child something it really doesn't need because this mom is going to be in every single day until she gets her antibiotic anyway.

The only time you get abuses of the system with people who have health-care insurance is due to ignorance. They don't have a medical sense about them. They've seen things on TV and they don't realize that this is not an emergency. A cut, is a good example. A kid can come in with a huge cut on his forehead. Do people know that you have twelve hours to stitch that cut up? Sure, you want someone to be taken care of right away, but let's face it, they're going to be irritated if they have to wait out in the waiting room for two hours just because a heart attack victim came in and got all the attention. They don't realize some injuries and illnesses are just as easily and effectively treated at home without a visit to the doctor. They don't realize that this is something that doesn't have to be treated right this second in an emergency room. If need be, you can wait a few hours until the doctor's office opens up.

We are a quick-fix society. Oh, we are. That's what frustrates people with coming into primary care and then needing to be sent to a specialist. Nobody wants to waste time in our society. Time is precious. They say, "Fix it! Now! Don't make me go someplace else and have to sit and wait for an appointment. Fix it!"

That's what happens with dieting. People come to me all the time and ask, "What's the latest thing on dieting?" The latest thing is, it takes a lot of commitment and a long time. And you shouldn't even ever diet. You change your eating habits for life, and you exercise, for life. But they still want appetite suppressants and quick-fixes and fad diets and that kind of thing.

All of us are guilty of not always trying to educate people and telling them there isn't a quick fix. You just have to go home and get well. You have to take care of yourself and get well. Nobody wants to hear that. They don't want to hear that they have to miss work. They don't want to hear that they have to go home and go to bed and rest. They want us to do it for them. So after a while you just hand them the prescription and say, "Here. Here's the antibiotic." When you know that the antibiotic is not necessary and won't make any difference.

There's a saying that, "A cold will get better in seven days with an antibiotic, or it will get better in a week without an antibiotic." That's really true. So much of what we see are cases where all we can do is help people feel better, but that is important to them. It tells them, no you don't have pneumonia or no you don't have bronchitis, or no you don't have whatever it is that they're worrying that they have. They get reassured.

A man came to me a few weeks ago with chest pain and he was really frightened. Naturally. He had a strong family history of cardiovascular disease, but then in addition someone he works with about his same age just died of a heart attack. He's a relatively young man, early forties. It turned out he had a hiatal hernia and gastritis. His esophagus was being inflamed by the stomach acids irritating that area which was causing this chest pain.

Additionally we found that his cholesterol was up, but his treadmill test was fine. Really he was OK. It was more the fact that he works odd hours and eats poorly and eats at fast food restaurants and drinks a lot of caffeine. He was really happy to make all of the necessary changes in his life.

Our health behaviors impact on us so greatly. People don't necessarily want to hear that. They want to come in and they want us to give them some medicine to fix them. It's like that Rolaids commercial. They knew the American psyche. "I like pizza but it doesn't like me, so I eat it anyway and then take an antacid."

Some people are afraid of getting cancer from smoking but yet haven't been able to stop smoking, so they eat two carrots a day because they heard that maybe that will prevent them from getting cancer.

L ay people are becoming very sophisticated about knowledge of high-tech equipment. So what do they do? They hear about CAT scans on TV, so they come to the doctor and say, I want a CAT scan. Then, if they don't get the CAT scan, and something goes wrong, then the doctor can be sued. Lots of things are impacting the costs and the care, and it's time the patient assumed some of the responsibility of rising health-care costs.

D rug companies have started marketing directly to consumers before they even market it to us. There's a brand new drug that just came out. It's an antihistamine. I don't have anything against the product, I'm just using it as an example. In fact my husband said to me, "What about this new allergy medicine. I just was reading about it." I said, "What new allergy medicine?" And he said, "Well, it's right here in *Time* magazine." So I brought that to the office with me because nobody had detailed me about it. No drug reps had come up here to tell me about it. Instead, what they're doing is they're marketing it to the consumer so that the consumer will come in and say, "What about this new drug? I want it," rather than saying, "I have a problem with my allergies."

I had a patient come into me one day and say, "I want a vitamin B$_{12}$ shot. I've just stopped drinking and I really feel kind of dragged out, and then I've been working really hard, and I really need a vitamin B$_{12}$ shot." I thought, no. I'm going to educate this person. I'm not going to do this. I said, "You know we give vitamin B$_{12}$ shots when there's a certain type of anemia that you need a vitamin B$_{12}$ shot for. Otherwise it really doesn't make any difference." And he said, "How about just the placebo effect? I'll just go for the placebo effect." He was so up front with me. I thought, yeah, there's a lot of that, but I didn't give it to him. I said, "No, it's not going to make any difference. This is what you need to do instead. You need to get more rest, you need to quit pushing yourself." It's like drinking another cup of coffee or taking speed just to keep flogging yourself to death. You can't do that kind of thing.

You can lose patients because you're not giving them what they want. That's frustrating and upsetting. They don't want to hear about the hard route, they want the short route. I've known of people that really feed into that and give the patient anything that they want. There was some "cocktail" that was made up and a patient came in and said, "Don't you do the cocktail? It's vitamin B$_{12}$ and it's this and it's that and it's the other thing." No, I don't do that. But there are people that do. To keep patients, you don't get people angry. It's easy to give people what they want.

"Cabbages"—coronary artery bypass grafts, bypass surgery—are another one of my big pet peeves. There's enough studies to say that they're expensive, they're traumatic to the patient, and you've got to do them again in five years.

I know that it's hard to get people to lose weight. Only three percent of people who start out doing it stay with it. I know that it's hard to get people to change their way of life, but why are we telling these people, "We'll do a bypass and that will fix everything"? What we need to say to them is, "It will fix it for five years and then you'll be back in here, in this same place, cut open all the way, and having to recover from a very major surgery."

It's a real high-ticket item for the hospital and the surgeon and the pharmaceutical company. It's a big money maker. And it's real costly to the system.

I counsel people on good health behaviors and I know how frustrating it gets to help people to change. But I don't think we should be saying to them, we'll do this high-tech thing and everything will be OK, when really it's their behavior that's going to determine whether everything is going to be OK. If they do a cabbage and they stop smoking and they change their diet and they start exercising and they take real good care of themselves, it will last longer than five years. But if they go back to all of their old habits because they say, "It's been fixed," then they'll be back in there again with the same costs.

I think, in general, people don't really have a total handle and grasp on what medicine can do and what the health-care system can do for them. There is only so much. Our doctors are magnificent, wonderful human beings, so they're limited by their humanness. But we do have a fantastic system of care, but it can only do so much. We've done a lot to hurt ourselves. I think that people just naturally assume that they're going to be cared for, they can do whatever they please and still there's going to be this ongoing system of care for them.

I think we need an enlightened lay people. One of the reasons that heart problems and strokes have decreased is because of the education and the health information that our public is receiving. However, cancer is still going up, and I think that's partly due to our misplaced value on rights. "If I want to smoke and go to hell smoking, that's my privilege. That's my right, protected by the Constitution." The secondary smoke may kill somebody else, but our rights are protected. If this person smokes, he may get cancer, he may not die right away but go on for years and then finally it's us that are going to have to pay for his smoking habits. It goes like that.

The three best predictors of longevity are all lifestyle things that we can do something about—diet, exercise and not smoking. Just simple things. More people nowadays are giving that serious thought.

15

OUR PRESCRIPTION FOR REFORM

With the inevitable legislative health-care reform package likely to pass this year, our biggest question is, after the bill is passed and after the media interest has waned (within a matter of days no doubt when the next national crisis suddenly threatens us), then what? Do we just assume that the health-care crisis is over because Congress has passed a bill and the president has signed it? How will we know if our health-care reform is successful? If access and affordability are the two primary concerns of the American people, what will be an acceptable level of access? How will we determine the reasonable cost of health care to an individual? In all the proposed solutions, we are hard pressed to find measurable indicators of success defined anywhere. Then there is the most important point of all: the final evaluation of success can only be made by each individual, a determination that can't be legislated.

Admittedly we are pessimistic about legislative reform. Now, we could explain our position by addressing the Clinton health plan point by point but we won't for two reasons. First, we believe that the final reform package will be entirely different from what has been initially proposed, making our commentary obsolete by the time this book is published. Second, we believe that the direction in which legislative reform is heading is substantially off the mark. As we said in our Introduction, all proposals for reform we've seen or heard are fundamentally flawed because they fail to address the root problems. Bad medicine treats only the symptoms, not the causes of an illness. It never cures, it only delays the inevitable.

While we are more convinced than ever that the United States has the best health-care system in the world, it is not without problems. Indeed, we see five areas requiring immediate attention. These do not encompass every failing in the system, but they appear to us as the most logical and compelling areas to begin the process of reform. The first is the economic abuse by a few providers; the second is the statutory weakness in the licensing, credentialing and disciplining of health-care providers; the third is the need for health-care consumers to assume more active responsibility for their health care; the fourth is the necessity for tort reform in medical malpractice; and the fifth is addressing the continuing deterioration of the physician-patient relationship.

It might be of concern to some that we didn't list the two most prevalent issues in the health-care debate—access and affordability. Why? Because we believe those are symptoms. If we address the five points outlined above, we'll see marked improvement in those symptoms.

So, how to go about it? In formulating our proposal, we were guided by three prerequisites. Number one was to modify the current system, rather than toss it out the window and start from scratch. Number two was to move toward simplification of the system. And number three was that reform should be a *process* of improvement, not a quick fix, not a temporary solution. With these in mind, we began to examine the five areas identified above and develop strategies to deal with them effectively.

In light of the testimonies of those we interviewed, there can be little doubt that unethical, immoral, fraudulent and unscrupulous behavior does indeed exist in the health-care industry. It is not widespread, but it is significant. This is not only an inexcusable injustice and assault on those of us who are patients, it's an insult and defilement of the majority of health-care workers who are honorable, hard-working people. Why should a small percentage have license to unjustly enrich themselves at the expense of us all?

There's a lot of talk about preventive medicine in health-care reform, but unless we attempt to "prevent" the abuses that the current health-care system ignores, and in some cases sanctions by indifference or protectionism, there will be those who continue to benefit unjustly at the expense of those who are least able to protect themselves. If we could substantially reduce the amount of unnecessary surgeries alone, we would save enough to finance our goals of providing access of health care to all Americans.

How can this be done? We suggest that all State Boards of Medical Examiners be replaced by one Federal Board of Medical Examiners that would set uniform, consistent national standards, and relicense all doctors every six years by written examination. Then, grant that new agency the authority to determine precisely what medical and surgical procedures each physician or health-care practitioner would be licensed to perform. Local hospital medical staffs would not have the authority to grant an unqualified physician privileges to perform procedures that were outside his or her scope of training. This would also control much of the abuse of power by the incompetent, the negligent, the alcohol-, drug- or psychologically-impaired practitioner. Every health-care practitioner would be held to the same high standards according to their education and training.

Next, mandate that this National Medical Board be responsible for investigating, prosecuting and disciplining all health-care providers who violate professional or criminal codes of medical practice. Offenses would be categorized so violations of the most serious classifications would result in immediate disqualification for individual practitioners, partnerships and corporations. It would no longer be possible to simply pay a token fine or move to another state and resume practice. The offender would be removed from the national health-care system for life.Then, within this agency, a special medical fraud and abuse task force should be created. This task force would address not only the consumer complaints, but would pay equal attention to those filed by health-care professionals.

We propose that two areas already addressed by the current

system be dealt with more vigorously by the new national board. First, we would require mandatory jail sentences for practitioners, partners or corporate officers convicted of fraud and would require that their fines significantly exceed the estimated dollar amount of their unjust enrichment. The second area deals with providers convicted of substance abuse. They would be subject to mandatory suspension or revocation of privileges, rather than merely being required to participate in rehab programs while their practice continues uninterrupted. Second-time offenders would have mandatory revocation of privileges for life.

All of these health-care rules and regulations would be incorporated into federal law, punishable through federal courts.

The next step toward reform is to consolidate, standardize and eliminate duplication of state, federal and private licensing, accrediting and regulatory agencies and creating in their place a National Health Care Accreditation Board. This would free the health-care provider from redundant reporting, the ever-increasing paperwork that prevents hands-on patient care, and would ensure uniform standards in all areas of health care. We've heard the president speak of the advantages of having only one insurance form for patients. If that's desirable because it makes health care more convenient and cost-effective, doesn't it make sense to apply the same principle to those who are administering care?

So far we've discussed measures that would fortify the ethical foundation of the health-care industry. Now let's approach the financial end. The goal is to decrease bureaucracy, increase the consumer's power of choice, allow free-market forces to work *and* provides access and care to all Americans. It sounds too good to be true, but we do have a simple, and we believe, workable suggestion.

Eliminate all current federal and state funded health programs including Medicare, Medicaid and Champus (armed services insurance), and in their place establish one agency, the National Health Care Financing Board. This would substantially reduce health-care costs. It would eliminate most of the overgrown federal and state bureaucracy and it would reduce hospital expenses by lessening expensive reporting systems, financial staffs and consultants.

This agency would develop a national tiered medical program that would establish the level and extent of care to be provided to a citizen, as determined by their ability to pay. Under this National Financing Board, we would implement a simple health care voucher system that would provide universal access to all American citizens. It would include allowances for basic health-care benefits including catastrophic coverage. Payments and levels of benefits would be determined by the individual's reported income on their federal tax returns. Everyone will be eligible for the basic voucher package, and those who wish to invest in more extensive coverage would be allowed to do so.

For example, the unemployed or the retired person would receive a voucher, let's say it's $1,500 for the head of household and $1,000 for each dependent. (These figures are arbitrary—in fact, most insurance plans do not charge for more than two dependents. Voucher amounts would be determined by the Board based on current premium costs for desired benefits.) With that voucher, the individual would then shop for the most cost-effective health plan offered through private insurance companies. The Board would stipulate the minimum requirements for those packages—basic preventive care, prenatal care, and catastrophic insurance would be provided.

Even the already insured worker would be provided with the same voucher and would be covered under the same basic benefits package. The employer or the individual may then purchase additional coverage to supplement the plan. The result would be that any health insurance offered by an employer would once again be a fringe benefit, an incentive for workers to stay with that company. Ability to pay and willingness to pay would determine more extensive coverage.

To avoid the problem of overutilization, as with first-dollar coverage insurance plans, our plan calls for a graduated deductible, based on income, that would have to be met by the consumer. Therefore, the consumer would have to take some financial responsibility for health care, however small. Second, we propose a deductible tax credit for the unused portion of the voucher. This would be an incentive to the consumer to seek out the most cost-effective coverage. For their part insurance companies would no longer be able to refuse to insure any individual. Anyone presenting their voucher requesting the basic benefits package must be given insurance. "Cherry picking" healthier individuals or refusing insurance because of preexisting conditions would be eliminated, thereby spreading risk more equitably.

The National Health Care Financing Board would simply draft the checks annually and then the responsibility would shift to the individual health-care recipient. That check would require two endorsements, one of the recipient and one of the insurance carrier. By requiring two endorsements, this would prevent the use of those funds for anything other than the stipulated health-care coverage. Because the consumer is administrating his own insurance, those costs would be saved by the federal government.

Under this system, universal access would be provided and basic health-care needs would be met, but the responsibility for selection and provision of coverage would remain with the individual. This plan would increase competition among insurance companies; it would help eliminate price fixing by government agencies or insurance carriers; it would help control overutilization by both the insured and the provider; it would standardize coverage nationally; it would guarantee access; and it would allow individuals to assume complete control and responsibility for their health-care choices.

The second critical duty of the National Health Care Financing Board would be to assume an active position in educating the public about its health-care options. Regional listings of insurance carriers would be mailed in the same envelope as the voucher. Those insurance carriers would be screened and endorsed by the Board to ensure that benefit standards are met. Some may still insist that there is a segment of our population that is incapable of assuming that kind of responsibility for themselves, so for those individuals truly incapacitated and incapable of choosing an insurance company, the Board would randomly select one if asked to do so. Because the basic benefits package would be standardized, this would not adversely affect the quality of coverage.

In addition, the National Health Care Financing Board would spearhead public education in preventive medicine and wellness programs. This would help accomplish a reduction in overall costs—its effectiveness would directly affect the cost of voucher payments. The better we accomplish this task of education, the slower the increase in the voucher costs of coming years. While promoting preventive care, it would also encourage all acute care hospitals to establish ethics committees to address the issues of futile care and "end-of-life" costs.

If this plan were implemented, it would provide basic health-care benefits to all citizens, but it would also maintain the free enterprise system.

Nevertheless, one thing this plan does require is greater responsibility on the part of the health-care consumer and recipient. An individual who is concerned about their health should be concerned enough to take an active role in their health care, which means taking responsibility for educating oneself, accepting responsibility for adverse lifestyle behaviors and being accountable for overutilizing the system. It means that we are not helpless infants who are incapable of making decisions about those areas that affect us most intimately—and health care is right at the top of that list.

Requiring consumer reponsibility would mean that access to repeat procedures would be limited to one-time treatment unless measurable lifestyle changes can be documented. For example, an individual who chooses to continue smoking, eating poorly, gaining weight and avoiding exercise after a coronary bypass surgery, is also choosing to forfeit their right for funding of a second bypass operation. These costs would have to be assumed by that individual. This would be a cost-reducing mechanism that wouldn't be based on arbitrary selection, but rather would result from the individual's choice.

Another area of consumer accountability is overutilization of emergency rooms by those without life-threatening illnesses. Admittedly, part of the problem is availability, and we would suggest that all hospitals and health system agencies provide clinical care in facilities designed to handle lesser medical problems—with an emphasis on the construction of facilities in the inner cities and rural areas. Once these have been established, emergency rooms would have the authority to refer walk-in patients to those clinics

designed to treat nonemergency patients. Insurance coverage
would be modified to apply only to the appropriate facility. In
other words, an individual with a cold could be treated in an
emergency room, but that would become an out-of-pocket
expense.

The next issue on our reform list is tort reform. We are bom-
barded by stories of crooked lawyers and devious insurance companies that have used litigation to their economic advantage. We
believe there is some truth in that. However, too often the health-
care consumer's role in malpractice terrorism has been ignored.
If the clientele didn't exist, there would be no market for malpractice attorneys. We believe that it is time for the health-care consumer to assume some of the responsibility for skyrocketing
malpractice insurance premiums. Too many patients walk into
the health-care practitioner's office already looking for evidence
of malpractice. Too many frivolous lawsuits are filed. We would
like to see malpractice settlements become the judgments they
were intended to be—compensatory, rather than punitive.

The scope of tort reform cannot be addressed fully in several
paragraphs, it would require another book. But because it is so
entwined in our health-care problems, we want to offer several
starting points for reform. As with our health-care reform proposals, we've avoided the most obvious solution—caps on settlements—because we see large settlements as a symptom, not the
cause. We are instead proposing modifications to the system that,
we believe, address the underlying sources of abuse.

Number one: A large percentage of legal costs lies in discovery
depositions and interrogatories which often produce little new
knowledge. In theory, plaintiffs are supposed to have all their necessary evidence before filing a lawsuit. They are not supposed to
file without all the necessary evidence in the hope that evidence
will be found later. Therefore, discovery should be limited to
allow for the request of documents and admissions, and, in
extraordinary circumstances such as the imminent death of a witness, depositions. This would substantially reduce legal fees.

Number two: As a deterrent to frivolous lawsuits, defense
attorneys' fees and other defense costs of litigation should be paid
by any unsuccessful plaintiff. As it is today, whenever a plaintiff

can find an attorney who will work on a contingency, that plaintiff assumes no risk in implementing litigation. In common litigation, defense costs can often approach or exceed a quarter of a million dollars. Plaintiffs and attorneys would be far less likely to initiate frivolous settlement-harassment litigation if they had to assume the risk of those costs.

Number three: The next obvious step—eliminate contingency fees entirely for attorneys in malpractice cases. (Lawyers making millions on malpractice will fight this one tooth and nail.) It is only the patient who requires compensation for injury and suffering, not the attorney. The result will be that attorneys will only be willing to take on cases they believe they can successfully pursue.

The final area of reform lies where we began this book—in the physician-patient relationship. A good place to begin reversing the current trends in medicine would be in revamping the system of education for health-care providers, in particular for physicians, and throughout medical school, internship, and residency, mandatory classes in physician-patient relations should be offered. Emphasis should be placed on the "humanness" of medicine. Medicine should once again be promoted as an art form.

As this is occurring, patients should be educated—not only in their rights but also in their responsibilities toward their health-care practitioner. They must assume an active role in their health care. They should, as a priority, seek out a primary care practitioner, not rely on emergency rooms, or assume that role themselves by accumulating a team of specialists from which they pick and choose. If we as patients make ourselves educated consumers, we stand an excellent chance of finding that "friend and neighbor," that physician or nurse practitioner, whom we can trust to manage our care.

16

HOW TO SELECT A DOCTOR

A doctor is a friend I wish I did not need;
I know I cannot afford, but I am glad (s)he is there.
—an honest patient

We talked with a number of people regarding how one should go about choosing a doctor. The reactions ranged from the serious to the sarcastic, from seeing who the local hospital administrator uses as a family physician to trusting "the doctor who plays the violin in the local orchestra. At least he has some redeeming qualities." There was the often-expressed frustration with the fact that it is so difficult to find out any solid information about the doctors in the community. As one person put it: "Most people can find out more about a car they plan to buy than they can about a doctor who may hold their life in his hands."

One hopeful sign is that closely held state and federal information on physicians is becoming slightly more accessible— although it almost always needs an interpreter. One person told us that "recently the federal government began collecting information on state disciplinary actions, malpractice payments, and revocations of hospital privileges for its National Practitioner Data Bank. The problem is, consumers are forbidden by law to have access to the data." Another person suggested looking through the court data published in the local newspapers regarding legal actions against area doctors, a monumental and probably fruitless task. More than one person we interviewed suggested purchasing a dart board and taping the Yellow Pages listings for "Physicians" to it.

While bedside manner isn't everything—indeed, an overly sympathetic attitude may be compensating for a lack of medical skills—it must be stressed that finding a doctor whom you feel listens to you is all-important, and this is, ultimately, an individual judgment. No matter how fancy a doctor's credentials, awards and affiliations, if you feel that he does not listen to you, does not understand your questions or complaints, then you will have handed over your right and your responsibility to be an active participant in your health care, which, in the end, is the only thing that will keep you healthy.

Now we offer a simple checklist in selecting a doctor or any health-care practitioner:

1. CHECK THE MEDICAL CREDENTIALS: Check the medical credentials with the county medical society. Although it is fashionable among the new doctors to break away from the local medical society as a sign of their independent thinking or going against the establishment, the county medical society usually knows the reputation of a doctor and it tends to jealously guard the society's name.

2. CHECK THE DOCTOR-PATIENT RELATIONSHIP SKILLS: Check the doctor's ability to make his or her patients feel comfortable. Is he a good communicator? Does he at least speak your language well enough to answer questions to your satisfaction?

Check it out with other friends and neighbors. A satisfied customer tells at least five other friends, but a dissatisfied customer tells nine other people. Your friends and neighbors can be a good source to check out the reputation of a doctor. Keep in mind that you are not necessarily checking out the quality of medical care you will receive but the way it will be delivered to you.

3. VISIT THE CLINIC/DOCTOR'S OFFICE: Before you decide on a doctor, visit the office personally. Sit in the waiting room and observe the following:

How are the patients welcomed or greeted?

How long do they have to wait before seeing the doctor?

Do they have a lot of forms?

Does the office staff help in completing the forms if a patient is unable to understand?

Does the staff speak your language?

Is the staff courteous?

Is the staff willing to answer your questions politely?

Is there a place for children to play while waiting?

Do they have child care if you are going to see the doctor?

Do they provide transportation? Some clinics/hospitals do provide transportation, baby-sitting services and a children's playroom.

Check also the location of the facility, hours of operation, fee structure and sensitivity of the staff.

4. DOES THE DOCTOR SPEND QUALITY TIME WITH HIS PATIENTS? Three things most important for a wholesome doctor-patient relationship are: TIME, TOUCH and TALK. Observe if the doctor spends quality time with you. Will he be able to give you the personal attention you need to listen to you? Will he spend time to talk to you to explain the nature of your illness, the course of your treatment and ways to prevent it recurring in the future?

5. ACCESSIBILITY: Some time health care is available but it is not accessible. Check out the office/clinic hours. Usually the clinic hours are designed for the convenience of the employees not the patients. Most government clinics are open from 8:00 a.m. to 5:00 p.m. with weekends off. If you find a doctor who is open when working people can access his services, then you've found a doctor who is sensitive to the needs of the clients. Consider the location, too. Many clinics are located in places that are hard to find.

6. AFFORDABILITY: Most insurance companies and employers have drastically increased the patient's share of paying for medical care while drastically reducing the benefits. Check out the fee structure.

7. EXAMINE IF YOUR DOCTOR UNDERSTANDS THE PATIENT'S BILL OF RIGHTS. The Patient's Bill of Rights has guidelines for selecting a doctor. Key components of the Patient's Bill of Rights are summarized as follows:

The patient has the right to appropriate, considerate and courteous care, regardless of the source of payment for his care.

The patient has the right to receive complete information regarding his diagnosis, treatment and prognosis, in understandable terms and language.

The patient has the right to information and education before undergoing any procedures and to know the name of the doctor who will perform those procedures.

The patient has the right to treatment permitted by law and to be informed about the consequences of the doctor's actions.

The patient has the right to confidentiality. All medical records are to be kept strictly confidential.

The patient has the right to have the most suitable care at another facility if that becomes necessary.

The patient has the right to know if the hospital is associated with or owned by another organization.

The patient has the right to know the type of hospital ownership. Is it for-profit or not-for-profit? If it is for-profit, is it owned by local investors or a national corporation?

The patient has the right to refuse participation in any human experimentation in treatment.

The patient has a right to examine and receive copies of the medical bills and to receive an explanation.

The patient has the right to know the hospital policies and procedures as they apply to a patient's behavior.

The patient has the right to a second opinion without fear of angering the primary doctor.

The patient has a right to change doctors. The discharged doctor will continue treatment until a replacement doctor accepts the case. If you are not getting better and you don't feel that the doctor is paying enough attention to your complaints and symptoms, get another doctor.

Once you feel comfortable with and have selected a physician or other health-care practitioner, avoid these common erroneous premises.

1. The doctor knows best in all things, and is beyond questioning.

2. The patient is seen as a deviant person who is sick, due to his or her own fault.

3. The patient is expected to be passive.

4. The medical staff expects patients to be totally dependent on them.

5. Being self-reliant is not seen by the doctor as being practical, since it requires too much time.

6. The patient is expected to pay whatever the medical system demands.

It doesn't end there. Selecting a doctor is a two-way street. You expect friendly, considerate, honest and professional treatment. As a patient, you also have some responsibilities towards the relationship. These are:

1. When the doctor is taking your health history or asking you questions, you must give complete and honest responses.

2. Let the doctor make the interpretation and draw conclusions from your answers.

3. Be completely and totally honest in answering the doctor. One doctor's office that we know of has a sign in the waiting room that reads, "Don't exchange your symptoms with other waiting patients. I'm confused enough as it is."

4. As a patient, it is your responsibility to follow instructions.

5. You have to protect your health by proper nutrition, exercise and rest.

6. If possible, write out your questions beforehand, so your time with the doctor is productive and organized.

7. Be on time for your appointments. Extra patients are

booked because of some patients' failure to be on time or show up for scheduled appointments.

8. Provide all the requested information for office billing procedures. Delays in providing billing information costs money because it results in even greater delays in insurance company payments.

9. Don't forget to tell your doctor what other medications you might be taking. The medicines that you buy off the shelf at the local pharmacy when taken in combination with drugs prescribed by your doctor just might kill you.

10. Take all of the prescription medicine as ordered by the doctor or pharmacist. Stop taking the medicine only if severe side effects occur. The amount and duration of time of medication is scientifically calculated, so don't change the rules by yourself.

11. If you are being treated by another physician or health-care practitioner, don't keep it a secret from your doctor.

12. Never hesitate to ask the doctor what you consider to be an embarrassing question.

13. Be as specific as you can be about your problem.

14. Don't demand medicines if the doctor doesn't prescribe them for you.

15. Don't demand diagnostic testing.

16. Learn the symptoms of being a hypochondriac and control them.

17. Never fear the worst. Wait to worry about having a terminal disease.

18. Be reasonable, fair and trusting of your physician. Don't expect to be made young again.

19. Don't, in any way or for any purpose, attempt to intimidate the doctor by threatening lawsuits.

20. While we have the right to expect the professional best, acknowledge that your doctor is not divine, he or she is a human being. They have their good and bad days. They are not the source of all knowledge. They will make mistakes. (With luck, only very, very, minor ones.)

Modern medicine is based on a relationship between the doctor and the patient and every relationship demands that both parties make an effort to build the necessary rapport. When you make an effort to establish that rapport with your doctor, no doubt it will be reciprocated. If it's not, it's time to begin searching for another doctor.

Once the "friendship" and "neighbor" relationship is established, the doctor assumes the "control agent" position. The doctor has more extensive knowledge and experience in treating illness; therefore he or she should be allowed to practice in the manner and method he or she deems best suited for you. The doctor is vested with powers to admit patients to hospitals for care, prescribe orders for nurses and other paraprofessionals to carry out the patient care, and demand that the patient follow the prescribed regimen in order to get well.

You, too, can contribute to the success of treatment. You are expected to admit your illness and express a desire to get well. You must seek help and demonstrate that you are serious in your desire to get well. You must cooperate and follow orders if the reasons for those orders have been explained to your satisfaction. You must be a participant in the health-care delivery system, not just a recipient.